Yoga Nidra
MEDITATION

"Pierre Bonnasse's *Yoga Nidra Meditation* is no glib self-help book about using modern yoga nidra—the practice of visualizing images, having awareness of breath, and remaining immobile while in a lucid, sleep-like state—for getting rid of stress and anxiety. It is, instead, an in-depth, wise, and elegantly written presentation of the philosophy and practice of modern yoga nidra as nothing less than a means of attaining a 'taste of Being' of Brahman. In this, the book itself is a kind of meditation—the kind that one may read at bedtime in order to facilitate slipping into sleep."

ELLIOTT GOLDBERG, AUTHOR OF *THE PATH OF MODERN YOGA: THE HISTORY OF AN EMBODIED SPIRITUAL PRACTICE*

"*Yoga Nidra Meditation: The Sleep of the Sages* is as much about waking up as it is about sleeping. Bonnasse shows us how to wake up from the sleepy dreams that dull our consciousness and keep our natural enlightened state concealed. He tells us that to go beyond the body into our awakened state, first we have to go into the body, awakening its sensations and breath. The awakened state of the body then becomes the river that takes us beyond our limited sense of self. This is an important message, beautifully expressed, and the author offers powerful, yet simple, instructions on entering the state of yoga nidra for ourselves."

WILL JOHNSON, AUTHOR OF *BREATHING THROUGH THE WHOLE BODY* AND *EYES WIDE OPEN*

Yoga Nidra
MEDITATION

THE **SLEEP**
OF THE **SAGES**

Pierre Bonnasse

Translated by Karina Bharucha

Inner Traditions
Rochester, Vermont • Toronto, Canada

Inner Traditions
One Park Street
Rochester, Vermont 05767
www.InnerTraditions.com

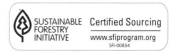

Text stock is SFI certified

Originally published in 2015 in French under the title *Yoga-nidrâ: La pratique du sommeil conscient* by Éditions Almora, 51 rue Orfila, 75020 Paris
First U.S. edition published in 2017 by Inner Traditions

Library of Congress Cataloging-in-Publication Data

Names: Bonnasse, Pierre, author.
Title: Yoga nidra meditation : the sleep of the sages / Pierre Bonnasse ; translated by Karina Bharucha.
Other titles: Yoga-nidrâ. English.
Description: First U.S. edition. | Rochester, Vermont : Inner Traditions, 2017. | Includes bibliographical references and index.
Identifiers: LCCN 2017029190 (print) | LCCN 2017011778 (e-book) | ISBN 9781620556771 (paperback) | ISBN 9781620556788 (e-book)
Subjects: LCSH: Relaxation. | Yoga. | Mind and body. | Meditation. | BISAC: BODY, MIND & SPIRIT / Meditation. | PHILOSOPHY / Eastern. | HEALTH & FITNESS / Yoga.
Classification: LCC RA785 (print) | LCC RA785 .B65813 2017 (e-book) | DDC 613.7/9—dc23
LC record available at https://lccn.loc.gov/2017011778

Printed and bound in the United States by Lake Book Manufacturing, Inc.
The text stock is SFI certified. The Sustainable Forestry Initiative® program promotes sustainable forest management.

10 9 8 7 6 5 4 3 2 1

Text design and layout by Priscilla Baker
This book was typeset in Garamond Premier Pro with Tide Sans and Gill Sans used as display typefaces

Cover image courtesy of iStock

To send correspondence to the author of this book, mail a first-class letter to the author c/o Inner Traditions • Bear & Company, One Park Street, Rochester, VT 05767, and we will forward the communication, or contact the author directly at **www.nidra-yoga.com**.

Contents

PART I

The Philosophy of Yoga Nidra

PART II

The Practice of Yoga Nidra

PART III

Putting Yoga Nidra into Practice

Four Practice Sessions and 115 Micro-Practices

• • •

Yoga Nidra

A Journey into the States of Matter, Consciousness, and the Joy of Being

Yoga nidra is an ancestral practice that comes from grand Indian traditions and philosophies grounded in Hinduism, Buddhism, and Tantrism. This unique form of yoga seeks to combine deep relaxation with attentive awareness in order to consciously explore the states of wakefulness, dream, and deep sleep. Moreover, it offers ways of putting the mind and the body to sleep while keeping the awareness alert. This highly comprehensive approach has inspired the discipline of Sophrology* and allows one to experience moments of great inner

---

*According to Wikipedia, the term Sophrology comes from ancient Greek *sôs* (healthy), *phrēn* (mind), and *-logia* (study of), and is a personal development technique founded in 1960 by Alfonso Caycedo, a Colombian neuropsychiatrist. It studies individual consciousness in order to allow a more conscious living. The term Sophrology has never been protected in its public use and resulted in many variations and divergences. Caycedo registered his original discipline as "Caycedian Sophrology." Sophrology in everyday use can refer either to Caycedian Sophrology or to other derived forms. Sophrology has its own methodology and original techniques, aiming to develop awareness in daily life and the autonomy of those who practice it. It is widely practiced in France today. (*Translator's note.*)

tranquility, joy, and well-being; one can directly observe particular physiological, emotional, and mental processes within oneself and understand them in a better way. By knowing that which is held on to, it is easier to let go of it and recognize the essential space of one's being, free from all states and processes. This practice combines very simple gestures and postures with light and subtle breathing exercises, as well as concentration and meditation, thereby allowing the alert observation of sensations, a welcoming of the phenomena that appear, and a return to the present moment, in order to taste the luminous and blissful presence to oneself and to the world, by day or by night.

During his research, Caycedo was guided by various traditions and currents, both Eastern and Western. Among the most influential for Sophrology were hypnosis and phenomenology, as well as yoga and Buddhism, mainly Zen Buddhism.

Practicing yoga nidra does not require any particular physical condition or quality, like strength, stamina, or flexibility. Simple poses (sitting, standing, and lying down) are used; they are adaptable to every individual and bring deep relaxation, as well as high quality attention and tranquility.

Through its positive, stabilizing, and pacifying effect on the body, emotions, and thoughts, yoga nidra is also a therapeutic technique that has considerably influenced modern relaxation techniques. Its practice reinforces joy, good spirits, and the immune system, thus preventing diseases, especially psychosomatic ones. It is the ideal practice for getting rid of stress, anxiety, and the fear of death, which yoga nidra considers to be at the source of all other fears.

By connecting Indian and Western philosophical ideas, and by drawing on the teachings of important spiritual masters, we will see how sleep can be an opportunity to practice a form of yoga that is absolutely delicious and that changes not only our nights, but also every minute of our days.

This book about the sleep of the sages takes us on a journey to the unknown and the mysterious, to the luminous presence of the unconscious mind, full of discoveries, encounters, and tastes; the art of taking a nap, a creative approach for lazing around, and another way of looking at life . . .

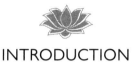

Indian Philosophy and the Limbs and Paths of Yoga

Truth is one, but sages call it by various names.

Rig Veda, 1:164–6

PERSPECTIVES ON INDIAN PHILOSOPHY

In India, sages believe that all paths everywhere in the world lead to the same mystery that humanity has never stopped looking for, whether we know it or not. The term Hinduism, coined by the British to label something that they did not understand, has no meaning; it tries to put the rites, practices, and philosophical schools of thought of this ancient land into one single basket that cannot contain them all. The term *Sanatana Dharma* is more suited, as it designates not only the myriad gods, goddesses, and practices, but also and above all the Eternal Philosophy, not as a theoretical discourse or an intellectual discipline, but as life support or a law of life itself, *what really is,* whether on an uncreated or a phenomenal level. This has nothing to do with an opinion. The term *dharma,* impossible to translate into our modern languages, refers to the objective law that reigns over the whole universe whether we know it or not. The concepts of social laws and moral and religious rules come much later, and are only a pale expression of it. This Eternal Philosophy is celebrated for the first time in the Vedas—ancient texts said to be revealed or heard. These texts, composed by the visionary sages of ancient India, divide knowledge or science into four parts. The *Rig Veda,* "the knowledge of verses," is the most ancient (1500 BCE). It contains formulas (mantra) and hymns and explains the Absolute. The Absolute is called *Brahman.* It is omnipresent, impersonal, and without form. The *Sama Veda* contains the knowledge of the hymns, or melodies. The *Yajur Veda* talks about the knowledge of sacrificial formulas. The *Atharva Veda,* the knowledge of Atharvan, is composed of incantations, chants, and prayers. These are followed by the interpretations and comments in the Brahmanas, esoteric texts called the Aranyakas, and the auxiliary disciplines associated with the study of the Vedas: phonetics, rituals, grammar, etymology, meter, and astronomy/astrology. But the essence of this revelation is crystallized in the famous philosophical manuals called the Upanishads (which literally means "to sit at the master's feet"), which are a finale to the Vedic canon, thus marking the accomplishment and the end of knowledge (*Vedanta*). They can be summarized in the four "great sayings" (*mahavakya*), related to each of the four Vedas, to be memorized and meditated on. The first statement defines the truth: "Consciousness is Brahman."* The second saying teaches us that the nature of our identity is ONE with Absolute Reality: "Thou art That." The third seems to be the statement of direct experience: "This Self (or Atman) is Brahman." Finally, the fourth, like a song of gratitude, realization, and liberation: "I am Brahman." Among the Vedic lords, let us mention Indra, the god of war, who is powerful; Mitra, the friend; and Varuna, the sky. These three are the custodians of order. Agni, the fire, and Rudra, the roarer,

---

*Respectively, *Aitareya Upanishad* 3:3 of the *Rig Veda, Chandogya Upanishad* 6:8.7 of the *Sama Veda, Mandukya Upanishad* 1:2 of the *Atharva Veda, Brhadaranyaka Upanishad* 1:4.10 of the *Yajur Veda.*

he who makes you cry shares many features with the famous god of the yogis, Shiva, the Auspicious One, mentioned in the later scriptures, as well as Vishnu, the omnipresent, he who pervades. And there are many others: sun gods, goddesses, demons, and other geniuses that mythology enthusiasts are sure to look up in the corresponding texts.

This Eternal Philosophy is also celebrated in the remembered texts (*smriti*) that constitute the entire foundation of the Indian tradition. These epics are among the most accessible texts, and are thus far more popular than the heard texts (*shruti*) known to priests, scholars, and a few spiritual seekers. The epics, while responding and referring to the authoritative revealed texts, speak to a large number of people through the story and mythology of gods and goddesses, imbued with a sense of profound philosophy. They include legendary and famous sagas like the *Mahabharata* (a subset of which, the *Bhagavad Gita,* is considered to be a part of the revealed knowledge) and the *Ramayana*. In these stories, the One, the impersonal Brahman of the revealed texts, takes multiple forms, usually more human and thus more familiar to the people, who in turn can easily identify with the manifestation (*avatar*) of Vishnu, such as Krishna or Rama or their companions. These texts also include mythological and religious collections that discuss the creation of the universe, the secondary creations, the ancestry of gods and sages, the creation of the human race and of the first humans, and the history of dynasties in a traditional manner. Most of them were written between the years 400 and 1200 BCE. There are also tantric textbooks, as well as books of law that mention moral precepts, codes of conduct, laws, legal treaties, penal codes, fixed by grand legislators such as Manu, who tries to reconcile the Vedic spirit with the current era. But dharma is not a dogma, and these texts were not necessarily followed, nor even considered popular enough by the British, who tried to impose a framework onto a reality that could not be limited to one particular setting.

For understanding this Eternal Philosophy or Eternal Truth, which cannot be seized by the intellect, the Indian tradition offers several points of view (*darshana*) accepted by the Vedic authority.

The *nyaya,* literally meaning "original nature," is the school of logic, founded by the ancient logician and philosopher Akshapada Gautama. It studies the means of knowledge, based on logical analysis and reasoning, by developing, for example, linguistic semantics. The *vaisheshika,* meaning "particular, specific," is a systematic school that classifies concepts; this philosophical and discriminative doctrine goes back to the first century, and it is traditionally credited to Kanada and his *Vaishesika Sutra,* composed of ten books. It allows for perceiving the characteristic differences between things. Its major ideas are of an ontological and systematic nature; the concepts are classified into six categories: substance, quality, activity, generic and discriminative substrata, and inherence. The *samkhya,* the "measurable," is the school of progressive discrimination of substances, credited to Kapila, whom some consider to be a manifestation of Vishnu. This point of view enunciates universal structures or the macrocosmos, and postulates a supreme principal, classifying elements into several categories. Yoga, which literally means "to harness" (*yuj*), is the exercise of spiritual communion, the means and the goal, the union with the highest Consciousness. Codified by Patanjali in his *Yoga Sutras,* the "king of yoga" (*raja yoga*) describes man's inner universe from the theist perspective of the *samkhya.* This is an integral practice, a means of inner investigation to know the Self, traditionally divided into eight limbs or stages (*ashtanga,* which we explore in the next chapter). The *mimamsa* is about hermeneutics, the exegesis of the Vedic ritual, other rituals, and ceremonies. The *Mimamsa Sutra,* exposing this doctrine, came after the fourth century, but is credited to Jaimini, who is also the author of an essay on domestic rituals. Finally, the Vedanta, literally meaning "the end of knowledge," designates the culmination of Indian philosophy in "nonduality" (*advaita*). This school is credited to Vyasa. It is the philosophy exposed in the Upanishads, made famous and developed by Adi Shankaracharya (788–820 CE), "the benevolent master" who lived in Varanasi, where he taught this direct philosophy. He is credited with numerous writings; he founded four monasteries, was the source of several schools of thought, and had an important influence and authority on this teaching of nonduality, popularized by grand sages such as Ramana Maharshi, Nisargadatta Maharaj, and Swami Chinmayananda. This path invites one to recognize the Self through three distinct forms of yoga, respectively involving the body, the emotions, and the mind: *karma yoga,* the path of action; *bhakti yoga,* the path of devotion; *jnana yoga,* the path of self-inquiry. The essence of these three classical forms of yoga is naturally involved with other forms of practice, and in the end all the paths come together in the space of direct experience.

THE LIMBS AND PATHS OF YOGA

In his famous *Yoga Sutras,* Patanjali enunciates eight limbs or stages of *raja yoga* that lead to the realization of the highest Consciousness. The first limb (*yama*) invites us to observe and cultivate five qualities, directly linked with our relation with others: benevolence or nonviolence, truthfulness, nonstealing, celibacy, and nonpossessiveness. Inextricably linked with the latter, the second limb (*niyama*) directly refers to our relation with ourselves, and consists in the cultivation of purity, moderation, or contentment; the strength acquired by asceticism; the knowledge acquired by the reading of sacred texts; and the faith acquired by meditation. Some may see this as a simple code of conduct, but the tantric schools prefer to set it aside for diverse reasons. That being said, these observances are of invaluable aid in cultivating the tranquility that is necessary for the practice of yoga. They are also, from another point of view, the fruits of serious asceticism. The third limb concerns postures (*asana*), the way of "staying" and the mastery of the body in general. The fourth limb encourages the control of breath (*pranayama*) by observing it attentively, as well as the practice of codified breathing exercises. These first four limbs are essentially related to the outer aspect of the discipline; the other four limbs will directly immerse us in the very core of inwardness. The fifth limb calls for the withdrawal of the senses (*pratyahara*), allowing the attention to come back, beyond the sensory levels. The sixth limb is concentration (*dharana*), the ability to maintain one's attention on a single point. The seventh limb, naturally following from the previous limb, is meditation (*dhyana*) and consists in remaining in an impersonal and equanimous observation where the attention is free and not oriented toward any particular thing. In meditation, the dualistic subject-object relationship is transcended, thus opening the door to the eighth limb, which is profound contemplation (*samadhi*), total fusion with the original Vision, and an answer to the definition of yoga initially provided by Patanjali: "yoga is the stopping of the fluctuations of the mind."[1] It is this suspension of the agitation of the mind—along with the help of these different limbs—that will allow for the unveiling of Pure Consciousness, of being, of peace, silence, and joy. Stopping the flow of thoughts allows one to experience the divine nondualistic reality in which these very thoughts appear and disappear. This extinction of thoughts, and consequently of the ego (the sense of "me"), in the vibrating void of awareness can also be that ultimate experience that the Buddhists call *nirvana.* Even though they are several types of *samadhi,* its reality is a matter of direct experience and cannot be understood through concepts.

The limbs of yoga cannot be limited to those mentioned by Patanjali. The tantric schools—which follow unorthodox points of view and do not necessarily answer to the Vedic and religious authorities—enunciate other components of the path of yoga. In addition to the first two moral observations, there are cleansing techniques (for the lungs, nose, intestines, and so forth), specific contractions, formulas, gestures, eye exercises, diagrams, energetic massages, rituals, therapeutic practices, and other interesting methods that are very precise and that incorporate the others. Yoga nidra is one of these practices.

PART I

THE PHILOSOPHY OF YOGA NIDRA

The Origins of Yoga Nidra

The origins of yoga nidra are lost in time immemorial, and one could also say that they are lost in the mysterious source of time itself.

For some, yoga nidra originates from schools of tantric Shaivism, and for others, from Vishnuist teachings; but we also find traces in medical publications and in many other schools, whether they are tantric, Vedantic, Buddhist, in India, or elsewhere.

In India, the Lord of Sleep sometimes takes the form of Vishnu, as Narayana, consciously asleep on the waters of manifestation; and sometimes, he takes the form of the king of yogis, Shiva himself, lying down like a corpse under the dancing body of the furious Kali. In both cases, the gods represent the Ultimate Witness that we all are, the Pure Awareness that the practice of yoga nidra encourages us to recognize, or at least make ourselves available to, by opening up to it.

Both these divinities—their names as well as their representations—can be used as important tools for our practice. Devotional chanting awakens the feeling and the form, makes us humble, and inspires us, thus bringing us back to the Presence. The power of images can help us to concentrate, appease us, and connect us with ourselves. The repetition of the mantra also allows for the recognition of a silent space prior to all thoughts. All these traditional practices bring the unique taste of the divine and the joy without object; and yoga nidra only helps us to lift the veil that separates us from them. Vishnu, in the aspect of "the abode of man" (Narayana), or Shiva, in the aspect of the "benevolent corpse" (*shiva-shava*), like all divinities of the Indian pantheon, are nothing but inspirational forms of the One that remains, who is also the Unique Teacher, life in all its manifestations, and because of whom we can learn everything, forget everything, and understand everything.

In the *Mahabharata*, the great story of India, one of the chapters mentions the thousand names of Vishnu, the Omnipresent, that the famous warrior Bhishma the terrible teaches to Yudishtra, the eldest of the Pancha Pandavas. As for the myth of Narayana, some see it not only in the impersonal origins of yoga nidra, but also in the origins of the world. Everything related to these teachings carries an instruction, which therefore by analogy carries many interesting indications for the practice and the attitude to be adopted. The literal translation of this short and poetic text does not do justice to the richness of the original Sanskrit text; each word in Sanskrit deserves a short commentary, so that one can relish its profound meaning to the fullest.

> I salute the Master of the Gods, whose navel sports a lotus, who lies serenely on the infinite serpent.
>
> Foundation of the universe, like the sky, like a cloud, with harmonious limbs.
>
> Lakshmi's beloved Lord, the lotus-eyed, who is perceived by yogis in meditation.
>
> I salute Vishnu, who is the destroyer of the fear of existence, the unique Lord of all worlds![1]

Narayana is not designated as such, but the description of this very particular aspect of Vishnu corresponds to his description. His name comes from *nara* (man) and *ayana* (refuge or abode): literally "the one in whom man finds refuge" or "the one in whom man abides." One could also translate it as "the refuge of men" or even "he who abides in man." He is also called Vasudeva, "God in whom all reside." His name immediately reminds us of the Self resplendent in all of us, and outside all of us as well, because he is everywhere, at all times. Narayana lies on water in the eternal state of conscious sleep (yoga nidra). He has four arms holding a conch, a disc, a club, and a lotus. The Supreme Master remains the unmanifested observer of the dissolution of the universe into the informal state of the causal ocean. The remnants of the manifestation have coagulated to form the serpent Shesha, who serves as a bed for the god. Also known as Ananta, which signifies infinite or unlimited in Sanskrit, the cosmic serpent represents energy, the universe's life itself, the vibration flowing in the axis of our back and in the very core of all our cells. This subtle aspect encourages us to unite (yoga) with the unchanging Witness of the phenomenal manifestations of the waking and dream states, which disappear at night in the bliss of deep sleep. Narayana is above even these three states, immersed in the bliss of the fourth state (*turiya*). Lying on his back, he remains happy and peaceful, in total awareness of this background of unlimited and infinite consciousness-energy, in which everything appears and disappears, where everything is born and dies, beyond even the very idea of creation or awakening, of maintaining or dreaming, of destruction or sleep. Thus tranquility seems to be a primary and essential quality. The dissolution of the universe happens through the dissolution of the elements (*tattva*), from gross to subtle, like the shutting down of the senses when one falls asleep. From Narayana's navel rises Lord Brahma, peacefully creating the worlds from his lotus seat. The representation of Narayana, paradoxical symbol of the unmanifested, has very powerful symbolism: lying down, asleep on the shoreless waters in the corpse pose (*shavasana*), he is contemplating, in eternal yoga nidra, the worlds appearing and disappearing within him, that do not affect him, thereby explaining his peaceful appearance that the yogi is encouraged to imitate and share. He witnesses the actions of the three gods of the *Trimurti:* Brahma, who Generates; Vishnu, who Organizes; and Shiva, who Destroys (together these three roles form G.O.D.). Thus he is beyond them all, *Parabrahman,* the Unmanifested, the Supreme above the supreme, and the Absolute Space that contains everything. The serpent is the bed (or the yoga mat) on which he sleeps. The serpent is not any ordinary one, and because it is carrying the Omnipresent himself, it is also That itself, like the Shiva-Shakti couple, signifying Consciousness and Energy. Here the serpent incarnates force, power, *kundalini-shakti,* the energy at the very source of all manifestation springing from Narayana's navel, by the grace of Brahma who is generating and creating the worlds and is seated on the pink lotus that symbolizes beauty and purity. As an epithet it refers to the goddess Lakshmi ("pure as a lotus"), Narayana's Shakti, touching the feet of her beloved—who rules over all gods—in order to make him feel her presence, just as the yogi brings his attention to his foot to become aware of it. Narayana is the pillar, the base, the support, the foundation, and the container of the entire universe and of all the worlds; he contains everything, he is omnipresent. He is not only what is happening, but the very space that allows things to happen and all phenomena to appear. He is the very space of Awareness; he is like the sky; he resembles it, is infinite and unlimited. Outwardly, in appearance, his skin is the color of the clouds. He is the essence of sounds and words, of prose and poetry; he is the flavor of everything. The limbs of his body are bright, luminous, golden, beautiful, splendid, and auspicious. He crystallizes positive qualities, reminding us that he is also happy, distinguished, honest, virtuous, and prosperous; this last quality is reinforced by the symbolism of the goddess. He is indeed the husband, the magnificent beloved of the splendid Lakshmi, whose name means "fortune," the goddess of prosperity and luck, riches and abundance. She is born from a lotus created by the churning of the primordial ocean of milk. She is often represented on a lotus-shaped pedestal, holding a lotus symbolizing abundance, often shown with two elephants. Businessmen in India invoke her as they cash in money from a transaction, or to ensure material prosperity. Narayana has eyes like a pink lotus, evoking the ten forces of Shakti and the eyes of Lord Krishna, the lotus-eyed. The yogis who practice meditation (*dhyana*) unite with Narayana (that is, they recognize him in themselves), in whom their fears dissolve. By practicing yoga nidra, by socializing with Narayana, imitating him, meeting him, and understanding him, the duality of desires and aversions will be surpassed. In Narayana, in conscious deep sleep, one finds rest and peace of the soul (*atman*). The last verse encourages total abandonment and surrender to the background of attention. I welcome, I salute, I pay tribute, I show respect, I praise, revere, celebrate, and honor Lord

Vishnu, to whom I offer myself entirely: not to an outer representation, not to a mere idol, but to the all-embracing consciousness itself, without form (as indicated by the root of the word *vish,* to spread, expand, penetrate, bathe in), that dazzles the world by the play of its projections, thus creating illusion (*maya*). The experience of recognizing the Self eliminates the fear, dread, and distress related to one's existence. Bhava, "Being," and Hara, "the Remover," are epithets of Shiva that dissolve the torments of birth, dream, and wakefulness in deep sleep, similar to death, which in Narayana is a mere concept projected by the mind. The merging with the One destroys all false vision, erasing identification with the multiple manifestations of the non-Self. Hari-Hara (who removes) also articulates the union of Vishnu and Shiva, as related in the *Skanda Upanishad:* "Vishnu is Shiva's heart, and Shiva is Vishnu's." The Lord of the Unmanifest is the grand master who takes all forms: he is unique, he is One without a second, the only One, the master of the entire universe, of all the worlds and phenomena that appear, are held, and disappear in him.

Similarly, we could also apply the same qualities to Shiva, the benevolent and the Lord of Sleep.[2] In one of his numerous representations, he is shown lying down under the goddess Kali, who is dancing on his lifeless body, after a tough battle:

> Intoxicated with the blood of the demons, Kali began to dance about wildly on the battlefield. The universe, rattled at its very foundation, swayed under her feet. All of creation could be destroyed by the goddess's frenzy. So Shiva, in order to save the world, threw himself under Kali's feet and absorbed the terrible vibrations into his own body. The goddess, having realized how much she was endangering the world, stuck out her tongue in shame, and thus regained her peaceful aspect of Parvati.[3]

Without energy (*shakti*), God himself would be nothing but a lifeless body, a corpse (*shava*); but this energy would not exist had it not been for this unique source of all life. The couple symbolizes the unity of all things, the surpassing of all opposites and duality of phenomena, as well as the recognition of the unchanging in the very heart of the moving ephemeral. In the practice of yoga nidra, Shiva is the motionless witness of the vibrating awareness in the body's cells, the tranquil spectator of sensations, thoughts, or images, and of all phenomena that continuously appear and disappear within him, at all times. In this legend, Shiva also appears as a child in order to awaken Ma Kali's, or the Mother's, compassion. This myth refers directly to our practice; with the attitude of a child who is discovering the world for the first time, without bias or prejudice, the energy calms down, takes charge, comforts, and nourishes. Be it in the corpse form or in the form of a child, Shiva awakens compassion and love. Ultimately, the goddess of consciousness is only cutting the ropes of illusion and the heads of ego that separate us from the pure joy that we seek in external pleasures even though it is already within us, in the mystery of the being.

This is why the mantra (or prayer) always encourages us to bow down to and salute, celebrate, remember, and unite with this Pure Awareness present in all of us, beyond the multiple forms taken by the gods and goddesses of India and elsewhere. Spiritual salutation, if I may use the term, encourages a transformation of vision, a coming back of the attention to itself, a presence to the openness and dissolution of thoughts in the Self. The rhythm of the mantra—be it *Om namah shivaya* or *Om namo narayanaya*—also expresses this dissolution and progressive sinking into the depths of oneself and of conscious sleep. The mantra calls for the energy flooding the background to unite with this "I am" knowledge, ever peaceful witness to that which appears and disappears. The very vibration of *AUM* encourages one to feel the manifestations of wakefulness (*A*), dream state (*U*), and deep sleep (*M*), which all eventually dissolve in the underlying and silent essence of the sensitive aspect of sound. Narayana, like Shiva, is in everything and contains everything; he is vast and he is expansion itself. He is the Self, the Consciousness (*chit*), the Supreme Being (*sat*) overflowing with bliss (*ananda*), which alternately takes the forms of creation, organization, and destruction. He is the great I, all-pervasive, beyond time and space, and beyond space and its contents; he is the grand master who teaches the seers the art of sleeping of the sages.

As for the term *nidra,* it has many meanings. Sometimes, it designates the act of sleeping or falling asleep; sometimes it refers to sleep with or without dreams, or it may refer to losing consciousness in the literal sense as well as to the disappearing of the mind or all attention.* But is also designates total awareness in deep sleep, in dream state, or in wakefulness; thus, it is no more than the very nature of Shiva or Vishnu. It is That. The term *yoga nidra* therefore directly refers to the union with this Presence; or rather, it refers to recognizing this Presence. For it is not bound by a common subject-object relationship, but rather refers to an intuitive holding, with no subject to hold. Hence, yoga nidra is both the means and the end leading to this. Adi Shankaracharya, the great master of nonduality (Advaita Vedanta), writes in one of his essays:

> Through appropriate practice, done steadily when all thoughts and intentions are completely rooted out, when we are freed totally from the web of *Karma,* then the yogi reaches and remains in the state of Yoga Nidra.
>
> Resting in the bed of the *Turiya* state, higher than the other three states; always having the vision of the highest; my dear friend, enter and remain in the *Nirvikalpa* state, the state of Yoga Nidra.[4]

Here, Shankaracharya reminds us of the aim of yoga: with the stopping of discursive and associative thoughts, certainty and doubt are immediately rooted out. With sincere practice, this quality of total

---

*In the *Yoga Sutras, nidra* designates one of the modifications of the mind, namely the state of dreaming, which is merely an agitation of the mind based on imaginary content, which the practice of yoga allows one to perceive consciously. In another important classical text of yoga, the *Hatha Yoga Pradipika,* the term is also used to designate sleep in the general sense of the word.

awareness, which he presently refers to as "Yoga Nidra," grows in the yogi. Opening up to the unknown allows one to encounter peace in this mysterious fourth space in which the states of waking, dreaming, and deep sleep appear and disappear. The aim of yoga nidra as a means is to recognize and understand all the manifestations of these states in a deep, alert, and equanimous state of peace. For in order to let go of something, one must know what one is holding on to. Thus, by observing and letting go of all phenomena, the yogi can finally enjoy this never-ending sleep, empty of all thoughts, whether he is busy doing something, dreaming, or fast asleep.

States of Consciousness

The ancient Upanishads acknowledge four states of consciousness: wakefulness, dreams, deep sleep, and a fourth state, which is the original unborn substratum, the very space in which the other three states appear and disappear. In this sense, it is not really a state that is changing and ephemeral, but the underlying reality to all states and other phenomena. In the practice of yoga nidra, this reality is the impersonal witness of the three states, the very Awareness that perceives the transition from wakefulness to sleep (with or without dreams), and from sleep to wakefulness. This Awareness is the transition itself, the very Ocean in which the waves rise and fall. The sound *AUM* represents this indivisible whole and includes all dimensions of time and space, although it is fundamentally above all dimensions. Each syllable embodies a state of awareness; and the three states, just like the sound and all phenomena, will end up disappearing, just like they appeared, in the silence of Pure Awareness. The chanting of *AUM* therefore constitutes a direct path to the fourth state, to the very source of all manifestation:

> They consider the Fourth to be that which is not conscious of the internal world, nor conscious of the external world, nor conscious

of both the worlds, nor a mass of consciousness, nor conscious, nor unconscious; which is unseen, beyond empirical dealings, beyond the grasp (of the organs of action), uninferable, unthinkable, indescribable; whose valid proof consists in the single belief in the Self; in which all phenomena cease; and which is unchanging, auspicious, and non-dual. That is the Self, and That is to be known.[5]

It is important at this stage to observe that true happiness, as described by these teachings, is not about making dreams come true, but just about realizing that we are, in fact, dreaming. And this is the case, be it in "wakefulness" or in the "REM sleep" state. In both cases, the mind is a common prey to agitation and suffering, identified with forms that it continuously projects and over which it has no control. As a result, one lives in illusion and associates deep sleep with total unawareness, when in fact in this state one is very close to abundant bliss, and therefore, very close to one's true nature:

> That state is deep sleep where the sleeper does not desire any enjoyable thing and does not see any dream. This third quarter is *Prajna* who has deep sleep as his sphere, in whom everything becomes undifferentiated, who is a mass of mere consciousness, who abounds in bliss, who is surely an enjoyer of bliss, and who is the doorway to the experience (of the dream and waking states).[6]

This is why Ramana Maharshi encourages us to be aware of our state of deep sleep in wakefulness: "Being aware of the deep sleep state while in the waking state is *Samadhi*."[7] This is also one of the important challenges of yoga nidra: to remain aware and alert, in the waking state as well as in the dream and deep-sleep states, while observing the unchanging in the very heart of the ephemeral.*

This availability calls for combining the most profound relaxation

---

Yoga Sutras 1:38. "He enjoys, but is not attached (on a karmic level) to his enjoyment" (*Mandukya Upanishad, Karika* 1:5).

with the highest attention; it calls for joining the peace of deep sleep with the total awareness of wakefulness. Yoga nidra will allow us to consciously investigate and recognize the nature and qualities of these different states, while questioning the nature of the "me" who behaves like he owns them:

> By piercing through the lower three states of consciousness (*jagrat, svapna* and *sushupti*) it becomes possible for consciousness to expand into the fourth state from which the lower three states are derived. The *jagrat* or waking state of consciousness comprises, in its widest sense, all knowledge when the subjective Self is in direct contact with the objective world around him on any plane. The *svapna* or dream state of consciousness comprises, in its widest, philosophical sense, all knowledge present in the mind when the subjective Self is engaged in mental activity in isolation from the objective world around him. The *sushupti* or dreamless state of consciousness comprises, in its widest, philosophical sense, all knowledge within the realm of the mind because it is based on lack of awareness of the One Reality caused by *Maya*. He in whose consciousness all these three states have become fused into one integrated state can wield all powers within that limited realm of manifestation.[8]

The "I am" Consciousness, the Supreme, thus pervades and is bigger than wakefulness, dream, and deep sleep, respectively associated with the physical, subtle, and causal bodies.* Before saying or noting that "I am dreaming that I am this or that," I AM; but because I am identified with the mechanics of phenomenal manifestation, I forget this and believe myself to be the changing and limited phenomena that I am not. Suffering begins when the spectator sees himself as the actor on stage and it continues until he realizes that he is not the movie projected on the screen, but just a witness to it, unaffected by what is happening on

---

*"It is one alone that is thus known in the three states." (*Mandukya Upanishad, Karika* 1). See the following chapter for more about the different bodies.

the screen. Thus, when I identify with phenomena appearing in myself, I identify with the world of objects (during wakefulness); the world of the senses, thoughts, and impressions (during dream state, wakefulness, and in the REM sleep state); and I identify with the emptiness of my own subjective world (during deep sleep), without noticing it. In other words, Shiva (I) manifests himself through the Trimurti (Am), by creating the worlds of imaginary ideas in the waking state (Brahma), by preserving them in the dream state (Vishnu), and by destroying them once again in deep sleep (Shiva).*

Let us note here that the tantric teachings of Kashmir Shaivism mention a fifth state, inextricably linked with the fourth, just as Shiva is inseparable from Shakti. Life is one, but it expresses itself in different forms. According to the tantric tradition, the life of human beings is not built around these five states of consciousness alone. Moreover, tantric belief asserts that these different states of consciousness hold the characteristics of all the other states within themselves. In other words, the Pure Consciousness, embodied in a body-mind organism, can thus identify with several distinctly different states, and this can happen in every state. For example, it is possible to distinguish a state of wakefulness in the waking state: in this case, the Awareness is identified with the objects of the outside world, such as physical bodies, forms, words, and names. This is, in fact, an absence of wakefulness in the true sense; a state of unconsciousness and total identification, in which I am completely identified with the material world, which is withholding all my attention. In the dream in waking state, there exists a form of awareness: I am completely identified with the inner world of sensory impressions, feelings, emotions, and thoughts. I look at someone, but I do not really see him or her, because I am immersed in various impressions, associative thoughts, biases, and representations of the mind. I am daydreaming; I am lost in my thoughts. In the deep sleep in waking state, I am unaware of the world outside and of the world of impres-

---

*A phenomenon appears, is sustained, and disappears or transforms itself. Brahma Generates, Vishnu Organizes, and Shiva Destroys (G.O.D.).

sions, because I do not perceive either of them: I am identified with the tranquil, impersonal, and blissful void of my own subjectivity, very close to Supreme Consciousness. In this state, the sense of "I" and "me" disappears, and consequently so do the desires and aversions that it generates, thereby leading to a state of rest and immense tranquility. Finally, in the fourth state during wakefulness, I am the Conscious Witness of the three other states that appear, are sustained, and disappear.[9] It is thus possible to investigate and perceive these different phenomena while remaining a witness at this observation post without thoughts, which is the fourth state. Yoga nidra encourages us to recognize it as being our true nature.

Who Am I?

Hence, it is about finding out who is the real subject; it is about asking the questions "Who am I?" and "Who is seeing?" and so on. It's not about finding out in an intellectual way, but rather in a direct way, through direct experience:

> "This body, O Kautenya is called Kshetra (the Field) and he who knows it is called Kshetrajna (the Knower-of-the-Field) by those who know them (Kshetra and Kshetrajna) i.e., by the sages.
> Know Me as the "Knower-of-the-Field" in all "Fields," O Bharata;
> Knowledge of the "Field" as also of the "Knower-of-the-Field" is considered by Me to be My Knowledge.[10]

In order to know the true "Knower-of-the-Field," it is first necessary to notice everything that belongs to the "field of knowledge" itself, through alert observation of its entire structure. When the field is noticed and dismissed in its totality, all that is left is the knower; and when the field and the knower are united in the light of a new perspective, that is Knowledge, says Krishna. It is recognizing in silence, and going beyond the one who thinks and pretends to know. To complete this inquiry properly, it is necessary to keep in mind that the "I" we are looking for cannot be, in absolute terms, an object of knowledge or something that can be seen or felt. Its mystery is beyond all experience, but is revealed during wholehearted experience. Perceiving the phenomenon in its impermanent and impersonal form reinforces the consciousness of the uncreated that reveals itself. As Nisargadatta Maharaj often said, "What was born must die. Only the unborn is deathless. Find what is it that never sleeps and never wakes, and whose pale reflection is our sense of 'I'."[11]

The Sheaths of the Being

The philosophy of yoga teaches us that the unborn, this "I am" beyond all sensations, feelings, and thoughts, is enveloped or veiled by five structures of different qualities. Each one of them says "me," claims to be this "I," appears, and then disappears by limiting itself to its limited form. But if I can perceive them, it means that I am fundamentally different from them.

Normally, when we say "me," we are first referring to our physical body (*annamaya kosha* or *sthula sharira*) and we are completely identified with this physical body: "I have pain, I am hungry, I am walking, I am sleeping . . . he is dead," and so on. In this case, I believe that I am the body. Indian philosophy, however, considers the physical body to be the gross body or the dense, material body, as a result of the solid and liquid foods that it absorbs. Identification with the gross body is clearly at its peak in the waking state (*jagrat*).

This physical body is enveloped, penetrated, and animated by the energetic sheath (*pranamaya kosha*), which is of utmost interest to us in the practice of yoga. It consists of the energy points (chakra and *adhara*), meridians (*nadi*), and vital breaths (*prana* and *vayu*). The energetic structure—which can be seen and felt, just like the physical body—feeds on the prana contained in the air. The mental sheath (*manomaya kosha*), even more subtle than the preceding sheath, feeds on the impressions received by the five senses. This is the inferior mind, composed of associative thoughts and memories, the ego or the personality, and common emotions. It holds all mental content such as knowledge and other memories. Beyond this sheath is the envelope of knowledge (*vijnanamaya kosha*), which corresponds to the capacity of discrimination. This is the superior mind, the intuitive body, where one can understand archetypes, symbols, and reality, without going through the habitual prism of associative thoughts. Along with the two sheaths aforementioned, it constitutes the subtle body (*sukshma* or *linga sharira*), and is active during wakefulness and during the dream (*svapna*) state. According to some teachings, it is this subtle body that reincarnates from one life to another until liberation, due to the impressions it has received (*samskara*), which have reinforced its dormant tendencies (*vasana*) of the desire to live and to possess, and these tendencies expedite the person's rebirth back into new incarnations (*samsara*). This is what happens every day: the "death" of sleep, the "reincarnation" at the time of waking up, and the reappearance of the sense of "me."

Lastly, the body of bliss (*anandamaya kosha*) or the causal body (*karana sharira*). It is impersonal, without form, and universal. It is the blissful space that we are usually identified with in deep sleep (*sushupti*). Being aware of the deep sleep state while in the waking state amounts to being aware of that silent state without thoughts, in which the sense of "I" and "me" has completely disappeared. In that very instant, there are no more problems; there isn't even anybody left to have problems. Each yoga nidra session is a marvelous opportunity to abandon oneself to the unknown, which we can profoundly and consciously experience and be, instead of just trying to describe it. We certainly do enjoy this state, but the practice cannot be limited to an act of indulgence. For if I am able to be aware of this state, what I am, in essence, is still beyond it (*turiya*).

The supreme body is none other than this fourth state (*turiya*), which is not really a state. It is the supreme samadhi, the unique witness, liberation, Brahman itself, the total extinction of the sense of "me" (what Buddhists refer to as *nirvana*), beyond all forms and concepts, beyond this stateless state itself according to Indian wisdom, beyond the fourth (*turiyatta*), and beyond Brahman (*parabrahman*).

With practice, yoga nidra will allow us to investigate, discover, recognize, and enter into these slightly disorganized structures. It will then be easier to navigate in these different sheaths or states, to try and recognize the sacred space or the Pure Awareness that unites, inhabits, embraces, and encompasses all of them. The union of profound tranquility with subtle attention or great alertness leads to this fourth quality of awareness. Let us note right away that this practice is not meant as a substitute for others, but can be practiced in addition to others. Therefore, it does not need to be practiced exclusively, and neither does it require any particular action. Although yoga nidra creates a context of availability conducive to recognizing Presence, it can also be recognized and cultivated while cutting vegetables, walking in the street, or talking to another person.

Awareness, Energy, Elements, and States of Matter

The tantric approach considers the universe and the being as the expression and expansion of the cosmic couple—Shiva (representing consciousness) and Shakti (representing energy)—that display the world of manifested phenomena in a permanent dance and embrace. It is as if the perception of one's own energy strengthens the awareness of one's own presence. The couple creates the world of manifested phenomena in order to recognize itself as pure bliss in its own creation. The human being obeys natural laws (dharma) that govern the cosmos. In Indian philosophy, there exists only one substance of vibratory texture, only one Absolute Reality, and that is Brahman, whose breath generates the existence of all phenomena, and who extends from gods to material forms. Brahman is thus present in all forms of creation and sustains the entire cosmos.

This manifestation of the being and the universe happens in two ways. Nature (*prakriti*), the dynamic feminine principle, is activated after contact with the static masculine principle, the Spirit, the Consciousness or the Being. This spirit or person (*purusha*) is the first reflection of Brahman, and is by nature free. This nature is the point of equilibrium of three essences, qualities, or behaviors (*guna*), on the basis of which each phenomenon manifests itself.

The energy of inertia (*tamas*), laziness, obscurity, inactivity, darkness, and blackness is the passive and negative force, the solid principle that mainly influences the physical body and matter in general, associated with the color black. The expansive energy of activity, desire, movement, fire, and digestion (*rajas*), is the positive, active, and affirmative force. It particularly influences the subtle body and is associated with the color red in the stomach region. Lastly, the energy of "truth" (*sattva*) designates the being, purity, essence, consciousness, the conciliatory force, nature's finest quality, associated with the energy centers of the heart and the throat. It particularly influences discriminative intelligence and is associated with clarity, the color white, and light.

The qualities interact on the cosmic level, as well as on the physical, energetic, and mental levels, by combining the five elements (earth, water, fire, air, and space) and their properties. This very energy is manifested through the evolution of the elementary substances (*tattva*). The play of these three opposite and complementary forces (as in the Tao) influences all individual or cosmic phenomena. Every phenomenon is the result of the five elements combined with these three forces. In equilibrium, they are original matter before its evolution, and their play unfolds all manifestation: as the forms become grosser, the vibrations become slower. Although inactive, *purusha* causes the development of the universe and the process of manifestation simply by his presence. The body-mind balance thus evidently depends upon the balance of these elements, supported by this presence and the force inherent to it. Each element contains the others in different proportions. Everything is penetrated by consciousness and energy. The malfunctioning of one element can mean that there is too much or not enough of another and this affects the body-mind structure; this is also taught in Indian medicine, Ayurveda, the knowledge of life.

Qualities of Sleep

Like all phenomena composed of the five elements and regulated by these three qualities, the mind's activity and sleep, which is a return to the matrix of life, also have different qualities.

Tamasic sleep is dense, without awareness, and may leave an impression of heaviness, stupor, and drowsiness on the physical as well as the mental level. In deep sleep, the stopping of the mind's activity is due to natural causes; it happens on its own, as opposed to in meditation, where an effort is required. Thus, it is not a yogic state of consciousness, but this natural interruption can serve the goal of yoga. Generally speaking, individuals are not even aware that they are asleep while they sleep. It is a state of total ignorance, unawareness, forgetfulness, and obscurity during which individuals recharge and from which they emerge invigorated, thus reinforcing the waking state, once they are "reincarnated" in the activities of the awakened body.

Rajastic sleep is troubled, agitated, and full of incoherent dreams involving the participation of the gross mind and emotional activity. If there is too much rajas in the heart center, as is the case in the waking state, the individual will be excitable, agitated, jealous, envious, and so on. The practice of yoga can then be a good opportunity to suck up this rajastic energy from the heart center and bring it back into the stomach region so as to harmonize vitality.

Sattvic sleep is almost dreamless, filled with a sense of deep contentment, with more lightness, awareness, and limpid clarity as of pale moonlight.[12] This impression can deepen and fill us with an even more profound feeling. Awareness does not completely disappear and what remains is this impression of moonlight in the dark night.

During the conscious sleep of yoga (yoga nidra), beyond the qualities and the three states of ordinary awareness, "the great sun is seen burning in the sky" and "what is night for all creatures, is day (time of waking) for the yogi."[13] The sensory system and the sense of "I" and "me" collapse, but the awareness is not identified with them. "I am" remains, bright and full of bliss, contemplating the rise and fall of sleep, dream, and wakefulness without being affected by them. Some Buddhists call it the sleep of clear light, or the union of vacuity and clarity. The body-mind structure sleeps but the awareness is neither lost in the obscurity of deep sleep nor caught up in the agitation of dreams; it remains in itself, in its purity, empty and luminous at the same time. This clarity illuminates the whole head, like the moon decorating Shiva's forehead, a symbol of still awareness and a witness. The body—the child—is sleeping; but the mother—the awareness—is watching over it. The illusion of separation, that an object exists separate from the subject, or that a distinct "me" exists, is dissolved. Only the Consciousness and the Joy of Being exist (*sat chit ananda*), inherent to the fourth state (*turiya*), to Brahman and to the Self (*atman*), which are all One.

The taste of this fourth quality of sleep allows me to clearly perceive the process of identification that makes me blindly attribute a personality to myself, limited to the body, emotions, and thoughts. It allows me to recognize that in essence I am infinite (*ananta*), eternal (*amrita*), unlimited, and without form (*arupa*). But, being identified with the body-mind structure, I confuse the form with the formless, the limited with the limitless, the eternal with the transitory, and I take the rope to be a snake. Nisargadatta Maharaj used to say, "In this reflection, the unlimited and the limited are confused and taken to be the same." And further, "To undo this confusion is the purpose of Yoga."[14] In this process, there is nothing to gain or desire. It is more a question of surrendering. Once what appears and disappears, what is born and dies, what awakens and sleeps is brushed aside, all that remains is what the sages sometimes call the "unborn," from where this Consciousness arises.

An Approach to Indian Psychology

The human being can perceive the phenomenal world, due to the light and force that illuminate, animate, and incorporate it. According to Hindu psychology, the immediate reflection of Consciousness is called the "internal organ" (*antahkarana*). It is composed of the psychic senses or the intellectual functions (the *tattva* of the psyche) constituting thoughts, and it is formed by the sattvic aspects of the elements. It is a structured whole called by different names that depend on the functions it performs. It is manifested on vibratory levels that increase in density. The intelligence (*buddhi*) is aware of what is perceived, records it, and evaluates it. It is the superior and impersonal intellectual principle, the faculty of perception, discrimination, resolution, decision, and intuition, beyond the sensations perceived by the body, and it determines the reality of facts. This reflection of the being is the inner witness. The sense of "me" (*ahamkara*) refers to the personality and the feeling of individuality that resides in the heart center, and from where selfishness, vanity, self-love, pride, desire, and aversion are expressed. Due to Nature's play (*prakriti*) and the qualities of energy (*guna*), I am identified and limited, and I react because I think myself to be the author of the action or the actor. Because I am identified with the body, I take myself to be a specific individual, separate from others, whereas only the body, the animated corpse, exercises this material manifestation. This identification creates the sense of a reactive and separate "me" and this sense of separation creates suffering, desire, and fear, consequently awakening beastly instincts. This "me" only exists from the mind's point of view, and it is nothing more than a mere thought, or a collection of more or less crystallized thoughts. Like the sun in water-filled vases, reality is reflected in different physical bodies, without being manifold. This discrimination, which consists in recognizing one's true and limitless nature, is the aim of yoga. The question "Who am I?" (*koham*) only aims at removing the painful thorn of identification, by dissipating the "I-me" illusion that the Buddha calls *anatta,* which is cause for much confusion. Lastly, what we refer to as the "mind" (*manas*) designates the ordinary associative thoughts, along with reasoning, memory, imagination, and emotions. The mind's function is to react automatically and unconsciously to the uninterrupted flow of sensations created by desire or aversion. Actually, the mind should only process the data given for the intellect (*buddhi*), but due to the sense of "me" (*ahamkara*), it claims ownership of this role. Its ceaseless activity provokes this sense of "me," which in turn sets the intellect into motion. The mind collects sensitive data, the sense of "me" measures its selfish worth, and the intellect evaluates and decides. But this discriminative faculty constantly interferes with the sense of "me," thus misinterpreting the received data, and consequently the perception of the world as it is. The Vedanta philosophy thus mentions a fourth internal organ related to the faculty of knowing and thinking (*citta*), translated as thought, mind, or consciousness, according to the context.* This is the part of the mind responsible for memories and the memory; it records impressions (*samskara*) and is like a reservoir. It is often considered to be the mind itself. The *Katha Upanishad* uses the image of a chariot: the passenger is the Self (*atman*) the driver is the intellect (*buddhi*), the reins are the mind (*manas*), the horses are the five sense organs (*jnanendriya*), the chariot is the body, and the road represents objects. It is a suggestive image to be meditated on in the light of self-observation.

---

*On this subject, I strongly recommend Swami Chinmayananda's talk *The Logic of Spirituality.*

The Manifestation of Phenomena

In the manifestation of this initial reflection, the phenomena continue to unfold on vibratory levels of increasing density. From *purusha* emerges *prakriti*, and from there emerges the internal organ (*antahkarana*) and its manifestations in creation. Following these essential elements or principles (*tattva*) of the psyche are those of the experience of the senses, due to which an individual makes contact with the manifestation surrounding her, through internal faculties of knowledge (*indriya*, the organ as well as the function) composed of the five senses (*jnanendriya*) and the five powers of action (*karmendriya*). Then come the five subtle principles or sensations (*tanmatra*), followed by the material elements (*mahabhuta*), which are the five elementary principles of matter composing all physical bodies. The five senses and the five powers of action are essentially animated by the rajastic force, whereas the *tanmatras* and the *mahabhutas* are animated by tamas. The evolution of the elements is produced under the influence of *purusha*.

The mechanism of perception operates in the following way: the five senses (smell, taste, and so forth) of the five organs (nose, tongue, and so forth) are affected by the five elements. This modification is transmitted to the mind that perceives, to the sense of "me" that reacts, and to the intellect that decides.

The practice of yoga nidra will allow us to understand these processes and their numerous interactions in a better way. The harness, the chariot, its horses, their reins, and their driver will be examined under a microscope, at rest as well as in action, under different angles. For example, we can do this is by becoming aware of the subtle sensations that emerge when we recognize the presence of the five elements within ourselves. Not only does such an exercise allow one to recognize the different states of matter and their interactions, but it also opens the way to the unconscious world of dormant tendencies, as well as to the very source from which these elements emerge:

> From that (*tat*), space (*akasha*) came forth: from space, air (*vayuh*) came forth: from air, fire (*tejah*) came forth: from fire, water (*apah*) came forth: and from water, earth (*prithvi*) came forth.*[15]

Matter, objects, and forms—subtle or gross, inner or outer—of the manifest material world appear from the combining of the elements. In the practice of yoga nidra, this is also a way of returning to and reintegrating the process of sleep, as well as in death. First, one must become aware of the solid principle and heaviness of the body, which is solid like the earth; then one must become aware of its fluidity and cohesion, which is fluid like water, with millions of "rivers" (*nadi*) flowing with subtle vibrations; then one must become aware of the body's heat, temperature, and glow, which are hot like fire; then of its movement and expansion, which are gaseous and vast like air. The aim, if we simplify and symbolize the process, is to become aware of the space element, of the void, the subtle quality of awareness itself, the essence of all the other elements and phenomena, and the very space from which they emerge and where they dissolve; not the physical space containing the objects, but the space of awareness in which this physical space itself appears. Thus, the practice of yoga nidra gives utmost importance to the observation of sensations in the body:

> All spiritual experiences correspond to sensations in the body. They are simply a closely graded series of different sensations, beginning with that of feeling oneself as heavy as a clod of earth and passing gradually, in full consciousness, to the sensation of liquidity and then to that of the emanation of heat. The last

---

*In the *Chandogya Upanishad*, *Tat* is the indifferentiated and unmanifested Reality that precedes universal manifestation.

sensation is that of a global vibration before reaching the Void (. . .). Each time a step is made on the ascending ladder, a sensation of expansion in space and of complete relaxation is experienced. This sensation offers a foretaste of what the experience of pure Spirit (*Chit*) might be, in which all things are transcended. (. . .) Yet at this moment spirit and matter appear to be one. This conception comes from an ancient theory of the purification of the elements (. . .).

Always remember that any sensation of expansion you may experience is a radiation. Remain calm and radiate this warmth. Do not question. Ask for nothing more. Live these moments to the full. This radiation is in itself *Shakti*, an instant of living consciousness, that is, a direct experience that is ingrained in you. Your sensation is the proof of it, a certainty you cannot efface from your memory.[16]

Such contemplation slowly but surely allows us to stop identifying with the play of the elements and realize that the alert and equanimous perception of sensations reinforces our awareness of the tranquil background in which they appear and disappear. This sheds new light on the following words of Krishna:

Weapons cleave It not, fire burns It not, water moistens It not, wind dries It not. This Self cannot be cut, nor burnt, nor moistened, nor dried up. It is eternal, all-pervading, stable, immovable and ancient.[17]

Such recognition first requires me to be totally present to the sensations in the body: not only in the tissues (skin, muscles, bones, organs) with their elemental qualities, but also and more importantly to the manifestation of the energy flow that animates them and breathes life into them.

The Energy System in Yoga

The energetic body constitutes the link between the body and the mind. It is inextricably linked with respiration, with the breath and its energy, omnipresent and always present in the universe: it is the "sheath of vital breath" (*pranamaya kosha*).

This vital breath (*prana*) has diverse functions in the human body, in the form of ten activities: five major and five minor vital breaths, whose balance—helped by the practice of yoga—is essential for the well-being of the mind-body structure. One can thus distinguish exhalation, the ascending function of the breath, closely related to the heart center: the breath of excretion, which expels everything and makes the energies descend, in close relation with the Earth, the anus, and the base energy center; the vital flow of digestion or assimilation, related to the stomach center; the flow of elevation, which plays a role in the rising of vital energy: it pulls up, elevates, and resides in the throat center. The synthesis of the four breaths maintains cohesion in the whole body and corresponds to the function of metabolism. It is the balancing and harmonizing energy that resides in the pubis center and in the whole body. The minor breaths are those that are responsible for belching, blinking, sneezing, yawning, and assimilation.

The vital breath of energy is subtle and circulates through "vibrant rivers" (*nadi*), known as meridians in other cultures. They fill, animate, and wrap up the physiological body in a circle measuring one and a half meters around the spine. Thus, human beings are constantly interacting with the cosmic environment through channeling centers, and these luminous channels are used for internal diffusion. They are woven into the subtle body, like threads in a net. Some teachings attribute them to the heart, while others attribute them to the base center, and the energies going through them circulate according to specific laws depending on numerous factors, such as solar and lunar movements, time, state, purity, and so forth. Their number varies: 360,000 according to some teachings, 72,000 according to others; but this is of little importance because everyone agrees on three main channels. The path of kind grace (*sushumna*) comes from the base of the spine, in level with the anus and the coccyx; it climbs up the axis, coming out through the fontanel. It is the royal path that the Energy of Consciousness (*kundalini-shakti*) goes through and the very path through which this life energy removes itself at the time of death. It is empty inside, with an underlying vibrating energy. The practice of yoga seeks to rub, activate, and heat this tree of life through postures, breathing exercises, concentrations, and sounds, in order to make it hot and vibrant. It is personified by Saraswati, the goddess of word and art. Surrounding her is the lunar or cool channel (*ida*) on the left side, which represents Ganga (both the river and the goddess that personifies it) in the microcosmos. It comes out from the right side of the groin, winding upward (or going up in a straight line) and encircling the energy centers. The left channel is pale, associated with feminine activity, with the left nostril, with inwardness, with death (which comes from the left side), and with calmness. The golden or solar channel (*pingala*) on the right side is a representation of the river Yamuna in the microcosmos. It is red and totally controls the external and masculine aspect; it is hot, active, and agitated, and it controls our actions.

Observation of ourselves, in yoga and in all daily activities, shows us how the energy circulates in these three channels. Breath will flow naturally in the lunar channel for an hour or two, depending on the individual, then in the middle channel, and then it will change sides. When the breath is solar, the air circulates more on the right side, and when the breath is lunar, it circulates on the left side. By intentionally purifying and rebalancing the energy with certain breathing practices, the breath will flow with more harmony and force. A new kind of sensitivity awakens.

The centers of consciousness, or the "wheels" of energy where the meridians cross over, are called chakra. They serve as regulators and transformers of the vital breath. The principal chakras are disposed along the axis and, depending on the school of thought, their number varies from three to twelve, of which seven are important. The other chakras are situated in the toes, soles of the feet, ankles, knees, and other joints of the physiological body. That said, it is important to keep in mind that a chakra never refers to an organ or a bone, even if one refers to them in analogy with the physical body.

The root support (*muladhara*) is situated at the base of the spine, at the base of the central channel. It is traditionally represented by a red lotus with four petals and a wheel with four spokes. A yellow square represents the earth and controls the sense of smell; it is linked to the feet and legs and holds the root mantra *LAM* on an elephant, symbolizing the terrestrial energies of strength, equilibrium, support, and firmness. It controls the physical body. The yogic tradition, sometimes difficult to understand, states that the Energy of Consciousness, *kundalini-shakti*, sleeps here, folded three and a half times like a snake around the supreme symbol of Shiva: an erect, self-engendered, and motionless sexual organ (*lingam*). Once this vital energy, represented by a red triangle, is awakened, it climbs upward, going through and purifying all the other centers.

Just above muladhara is the seat of the Self (*svadhisthana*), situated in level with the genitals and the sacrum. It is represented by a lotus with six red petals. A crescent represents the water element and it carries the sound *VAM,* resting on a crocodile-like creature. It controls the sense of taste. It is the psychic center of bliss and is related to the action of taking or to the hands. Vishnu is seated there on his throne, which is the eagle Garuda, he who devours.

Further up the axis, situated in level with the solar plexus, the center that is abundant with joy (*manipura*), is represented by a blue lotus with ten petals. In the middle, an inverted red triangle represents the fire element (from which jewels burst forth), and it carries the sound *RAM*, resting on a bull. It controls the sense of sight (no light without fire, and vice versa) and digestion. It is linked to the stomach, the eyes, the anus, the big toes, the spine, and all other fire points. Rudra, the tormentor, the furious, he who makes one cry, an epithet of Agni and a Vedic prototype of Shiva, lives here, covered in ashes and seated on a happy or joyous cow (*nandi*).

The energy center of the heart (*anahata*) is represented by a lotus with twelve golden petals. The air element is symbolized by two interlaced triangles (or a hexagon) and it carries the sound *YAM*; Isha is seated on a black antelope, symbolizing movement and rapidity. In the hexagon is an inverted triangle in which the *shivalingam* is resplendent, like a block of gold, a symbol of sexual desire. It is the seat of the individual soul and life, symbolized by a flame, motionless in space without the slightest breath of wind. From it emanates a subtle unbeaten sound (*anahata shabda*) that is born in silence. This sound relates to the sense of touch, the skin, sexual organs, respiration, and sleep. All the other senses owe their existence to it, and not the other way around, because contact is necessary for the perception of the senses. Another center also resides there, with eight petals, the wheel of felicity, where the devotee can represent his favorite deity under a magnificent wish tree, or even a gleaming heart surrounded by flames, like in the vision of Marie Alacoque, known as the Sacred Heart. Depending on the context, the heart refers to the actual organ, or the energy center, the Self or Pure Awareness, in which everything appears and disappears.

Situated at the level of the larynx, at the base of the throat and the cervical spine, the very pure center (*vishuddha*) is represented by a lotus with sixteen purple petals. A white circle in a triangle represents ether, the space element, shining like the full moon. It carries the sound *HAM,* resting on an elephant. It controls the sense of hearing. It is the center of the Sacred Verb, of manifested speech, in relation with the ears, the vocal cords, and the ascending vital breath. Shiva, in his androgynous form, dominates it. According to certain tantric texts, the awakening of this center brings liberation, allowing one to see the three forms of time and even beyond time.

Situated between the eyebrows, the commanding center (*ajna*) is represented by a white lotus with two petals. A white triangle symbolizes the mind and carries the sound *AUM*. It controls the mind and is the center of authority. It is the orchestra conductor of the other wheels of energy, the mental space in which the world appears. Here, Shiva resides in his phallic form, within a triangle symbolizing the feminine sexual organ.

Lastly, the center of a "thousand petals" (*sahasrara*) is situated at the "threshold of the divine," at the top of the occiput, at the back of the head, just above the fontanel. It is the abode of Shiva, whiter than the full moon, and symbolizes the final stage of realization. This thousand-petaled lotus of gold holds the fifty letters of the Sanskrit alphabet. In the middle of the lotus is a triangle, whose center holds the great void, symbol of supreme light and divine union. It is in fact outside the structure of the wheels of energy because if we compare the central channel to a road, the road does not even go there. Shiva is seated on a swan (*hamsa*), symbol of inhalation (*ham*) and exhalation (*sa*) signifying "I am (That)," the breath of Brahma, responsible for the creation and dissolution of the worlds. It is in this Absolute Void that the Energy of Consciousness ends its race and is dissolved, a symbol of the blissful union of Shiva and Shakti, representing Consciousness and Energy.

The energetic structure communicates with the physical and mental bodies through supports (*adhara*) or receptacles, where important information—necessary for all energetic and therapeutic practices—is exchanged. Yoga nidra will thus insist on the awareness and feeling of specific points in the big toes, ankles, knees, hips, inner and outer anal sphincters, the base of the sexual organs, between the pubis and the navel, in the solar plexus, the central point of the heart, the throat, uvula, occiput, the base of the tongue, the space between the eyebrows, the tip of the nose, the center of the head in the inner region of the forehead, and in the fontanel.

Let us also note the presence of certain "knots" (*granthi*) in the energetic structure. In the beginning, all individuals have three knots that characterize the human species. One of the goals of yoga is to understand and undo these three knots. Everyone must undo them in their lifetime in order to transcend the conditioning of the human species and accomplish their spiritual destiny. The knots are related to the three principle centers (chakra) in which the energies are the most powerful, as well as to the three gods of the Hindu trinity, symbolizing the generation, organization, and destruction of all phenomena. In the base energy center, the knot of creation expresses the animal, bodily, and sexual personalities. It can free the individual of animality, and in this way the body becomes a temple. In the heart center is situated the knot of the psychological personality and the ego, the space in which the individual is imprisoned in predetermined conditioning, heredity, and emotions. In the forehead center, the knot of reason and intelligence reinforces identification with the mind and with thoughts, but opens up to awareness when it is undone and when the mind's activities are stopped.

The Phenomenal World and Constructions of the Mind

From Socrates to Montaigne, philosophers teach us that the problem does not lie in reality itself, but in the way in which we perceive it. For millennia yoga has shown us why this happens, by confronting us with the mechanical part of ourselves that we often mistake for our true nature. When it is clearly seen that the objects and beings of the world only exist because they can be perceived, and when it is truly felt that they only constitute a vast network of sensations and thoughts, it can then be possible to let a positive and conscious influence be exercised on it. As soon as I stop taking the rope to be a snake, I am no longer afraid to grab onto it and use it in a good way. But the nature of the mind's processes expressed through consciousness, unconsciousness, and understanding makes me constantly go from apprehending reality to forgetting it. Yoga nidra allows me to understand that the more aware I am in sleep, the more aware I am in wakefulness, and vice versa. Knowing this can allow us to take a step back in the face of the automatic reactions of the mind-body structure. It also allows us to enrich the quality of our relation with ourselves and with the world, to find beauty in the most ordinary things by opening up to more beauty, joy, and flavor.

The Unconscious Mind

An alert and equanimous observation of the phenomena of sensations, emotions, and thoughts allows one to progressively open up to the dormant tendencies that condition them. Little by little, the practice can break down the natural barrier that exists between the conscious and the unconscious. The light of consciousness comes into our darkest places. It is impossible for us to understand the meaning of our present lives without becoming fully aware of all the phenomena that condition it. All impressions (*samskara*) that we receive at every moment of our lives leave imprints in us, they are the residual tendencies that mechanically condition our thoughts, words, actions (*karma*), and basically our whole life. When I react with desire or aversion to a sensation, I automatically create a new impression of desire or aversion that adds itself to the existing stock, thus strengthening my usual manner of thinking and reacting. In this way, I cultivate my suffering, remaining torn between the search for pleasure and pain.

Yoga offers many ways to eradicate and transcend this. During meditation, when the mind is deprived of the habitual flow of thoughts it will draw on its reserves, like a physical body when it is deprived of food. The deeply rooted impressions will then surface in the form of sensations and thoughts; but simply being aware of them and not reacting to them allows for their eradication because we are breaking the habitual mechanism of desire and aversion, which is the very source of our suffering. The path of selfless service (*seva*) is also a way to purify these tendencies: by serving others I can free myself of the selfish desires that generally motivate most of my actions. In fact, it is not the action in itself that creates new conditioning, but the attachment to the action and its result.* This is why the task of purifying the unconscious depends less on my actions and more on the inner attitude with which I accomplish and observe them. And it is the same for all other practices, be they physical, devotional, or contemplative.

The term *vasana* (the root is *vasa,* meaning "scent") can be translated as memory, desire, inclination, tendency, or illusion. It refers to the underlying tendency of our behavior, nourished by our past actions and the impressions we have received. It refers to the profound tendencies of our personality, and their "scent," which influences the mind without us realizing it. Ordinary awareness is a tumultuous flow of thoughts, ideas, and images. All psychological experiences are only mental agitations (*vritti*) that come from the perception of the senses and the expression of our dormant tendencies. Each desire leaves an imprint on the mind. These impregnations are manifested, for example, in the form of irresistible impulses and conditioned or uncontrolled reactions. The mind's life, during wakefulness and in dreams, is a continuous discharge of these profound tendencies and of the residual impressions of past sensations. Moment after moment, the mind refreshes this unconscious causal space, thus conditioning the specific character and personality of each individual. These dormant predispositions of the mind are also transferred through heredity or reincarnation. They nourish the desire to live, the feeling of existence (but not of Being), as well as the repetition of the same patterns of suffering going round and round in circles (*samsara*), obeying universal laws. They continue to live in the mind, conditioning us in such a way that their effects continue beyond their initial causes. They thus designate a factor of extension and of continuity, but also of intelligibility in space and time. These residual impressions nourish our memories and dreams, allowing for connections between specific phenomena at the same time. This is why, over

*This is one of the important teachings of the *Bhagavad Gita.*

and above the limitations and conditioning that they generate, they can be regarded as a force having some use in life.

In dreams as well as in our memory, the mind's content remains conditioned by these unconscious tendencies, although it is free from the influence of the sense organs. Dreams seem to be more complex than memories. While the latter essentially depend solely upon experiences, limiting them to the past (to the memory and to a conditioned personality), dreams benefit from a greater freedom of creativity due to the imaginary space, although they are conditioned by residual impressions and seem to be very real and consistent. Dreams originate from many diverse factors. They can be set off by the manifestation of an impression received before falling asleep, and this may give it a specific impulse or color. In this way, dreams reproduce a past experience of the state of wakefulness, but they can also be impressions of things experienced during the dream itself. The dream can also be triggered by some disturbance in the organism. And finally, in a more mysterious way, dreams can be triggered by the invisible plot of our destiny, by the invisible effects woven by our past actions, which allow us to see positive or negative situations and give a specific meaning to the dream. In this case, intuition is involved.

Beyond the role of purification that it accomplishes, the attitude of the witness or of the silent spectator reunites and links dreams with memories, thus reconciling all phenomena. But mostly, it allows one to open up to the sacred dimension beyond these two, for it is important to understand that neither dreams nor memories can awaken me to my true nature. They can help me to understand daily and phenomenal life a little better, with its desires and aversions, joys and sorrows. But I cannot really know myself in an absolute way through the immediate memory of the mind, through dreams, or through the profound memory related to dormant tendencies and impressions. Transcending the duality of the phenomenal world is not about making an effort, thinking, or performing an action; it is not related to memory or to time or space; and it is not about doing anything. It is more about an attitude of openness and availability, of effacement and surrender. The secret lies in relishing the luminous presence to oneself, in the pure consciousness of being, as I unconditionally listen to what is, here and now; because everything appears and disappears in this listening, without ever affecting it and troubling the profound silence inherent to it. Yoga nidra allows me to recognize this fundamental difference between what is taking place and the very space in which it occurs. Everything resides in a specific quality of attention that is completely impersonal:

> The discovery of your real nature cannot come about through memory. It comes through multidimensional attention, which occurs, naturally when memory is absent. This innate attention is listening. When you are in listening you feel yourself in vastness, in immensity where there is no listener or looker. Only in listening.[18]

Fears, Desires, and Suffering

All human beings desire happiness and feel aversion for suffering. In one way or another, they all look for happiness and try to escape misery. But alert observation reveals that the more I look for happiness, the more I distance myself from it. Absorbed in the dance of phenomena, I ignore my true nature—I take myself to be a separate entity and think that I am the author of my actions. Conditioned by dormant tendencies, I identify with names and forms and live in the illusion of existing as an individual. The mind and sense organs come into contact with objects, and each contact gives rise to a sensation. In my agitation, I react with desire or aversion to each one of these sensations without even realizing it. In this way, I collect impressions and accumulate imprints that continue to condition this mind-body structure that I call me. Gesticulating, blind and deaf, I go after what I like and try to avoid or escape what I don't like. In this way, I spend my time being discontent, reacting to the fact that what I do not desire happens to me and what I desire does not happen; this reinforces attachment to everything I think I own, and consequently, I fear that I will lose it. I wake up every morning and repeat the same pattern of desire, aversion, and sorrow, as I am caught up in the whirlwind of thoughts about what will happen, torn between the past and the future. I move, in this way, from one suffering to another, from youth to decrepitude, until I disappear into deep sleep or death.

Once again, it is not the actions themselves that nourish the stock of conditioning imprints and my suffering, but my personal and selfish attitude, motivated by the desire of gratification and recognition with which I accomplish these actions. A closer look at this selfishness shows that it is not even a deliberate and conscious choice, but it arises from a continuous flow of automatic thoughts with which I am completely identified and, in a matter of speaking, I am reduced to:

> When man thinks of objects, "attachment" for them arises; from attachment "desire" is born; from desire arises "anger" . . .
>
> From anger comes "delusion"; from delusion "loss of memory"; from loss of memory the "destruction of discrimination"; from destruction of discrimination, he "perishes."[19]

No one existing as a mind-body structure knows how to escape this tenacious mechanism. An ancient Sanskrit proverb says, substantially and poetically, that "the arrows of suffering that will pierce our hearts are equal to the number of our attachments." In other words, the suffering that is experienced is directly proportional to the attachment that we feel toward what is dear to us, starting with me and followed by what is mine.

To be free of suffering obviously does not mean that one should abstain from having friends and family, or feelings, or that one should be in denial of pain related to illness or sorrow related to mourning. I must realize that the vision that perceives this suffering is, by nature, distinct and free from it. In other words, I am not this suffering, because it appears and disappears in the consciousness that remains unaffected by what occurs in it. It is the awareness that I am.

So, looking for happiness comes down to seeking oneself, doesn't it? The absolute nature of the being and the absolute nature of consciousness and bliss are one and the same, aren't they? Trying to understand what I really am, or trying to think about happiness, is like looking for darkness with a flashlight. But desiring it or looking for it is not good or bad in itself. If I desire happiness, it is because some part of me has known it or knows it. So in that case, what is keeping me away from it? In deep sleep, I can recognize that there are no more problems, nor any solutions, and no me who thinks that he has any problems or solutions. In that very moment, I am immersed in profound bliss; I am, by nature, without desires or aversions. When I wake up, I identify with the body and the thoughts, I have new desires, and I suffer in consequence. Through repeated observation, I come to the conclusion that identification alone makes me suffer, and that having desire is not a hindrance, but a natural process that offers the possibility to *remember* that I am different from desire, every single time it arises. By paying attention to the desires that appear, I can open up to the joyous space of awareness in which they appear. In the same way, I can see that I aspire to be free only in the state of wakefulness. In deep sleep, or in the simple joy of being, this aspiration does not exist; it appears only with thought, and yet, everything is only joy and vastness. By looking for happiness or some kind of realization I only increase suffering. But when I am without ego, when "I-me" is suspended, like in an accident or during a nap or a yoga nidra session, a feeling of immense peace reminds me that it was always there:

> One does not aspire for Realization in deep sleep; the aspiration only arises in the waking state; the functions of the waking state are those of the ego that is fundamentally the "I." By discovering what this "I" is, and remaining as "I" (without the intention of doing anything), all doubts disappear. . . . Bring about sleep even in the

waking state and that is realization. Effort is directed to extinguishing the "I-thought" and not for ushering the true "I." For the latter is eternal and requires no effort on your part.[20]

Sleep and Death

By bringing us face to face with our sleep and making us lie down in the corpse pose, yoga nidra also brings us face to face with death. There can be no wakefulness without sleep, no life without death; and it is impossible for us to understand the nature of one state without understanding the nature of the other one. I am born and wake up as I inhale; I die and fall asleep as I exhale, in the pause after exhaling. It is not a simple coincidence that Hypnos and Thanatos are brothers in Greek mythology. Sleep can be considered preparation for death and a way to be free of the fear that death awakens:

> It is not without reason we are taught to take notice of our sleepe for the resemblance it hath with death. How easily we pass from waking to sleeping; with how little interest we lose the knowledge of light and of our selves. The facultie of sleepe might haply seeme unprofitable and against nature, sithence it depriveth up of all actions and barreth us of all sense, were it not that nature doth thereby instruct us that she hath equally made us as well to live as to die; and by life presenteth the eternal state unto us which she after the same reserveth for us, so to accustome us thereunto, and remove the feare of it from us.[21]

We all enjoy deep sleep and we even court it, and yet we remain prisoners of the fear of death. But I can realize that this fear appears only with the appearing of my thoughts and the sense of "me," in wakefulness and in dreams; and moreover, this fear disappears, no matter the state and the means, when my thoughts are stopped:

The ego is the same in wakefulness, dream and sleep. Find out the underlying Reality behind these states. That is the Reality underlying these. In that state, there is Being alone. There is no you, nor I, nor he; no present, nor past, nor future. It is beyond time and space, beyond expression. . . . If you understand waking and sleeping in their essence, you will understand life and death; the only difference is that waking up and going to sleep happens every day. . . . The dead are indeed happy. They have got rid of the troublesome overgrowth—the body. The dead man does not grieve. The survivors grieve for the man who is dead. Do men fear sleep? On the contrary, sleep is courted and on waking up every man says that he slept happily. One prepares the bed for sound sleep. Sleep is temporary death. Death is longer sleep.[22]

Yoga nidra invites us to become aware of the process of falling asleep, instead of experiencing it without awareness, every time the body is about to fall asleep, be it in bed at night, during a nap, or during exercises practiced during the day. However, we must understand that knowing is not enough. One must always renew the experience, as if for the very first time, without bias or prejudice; and also as if it were the very last time, as if each exhalation were the last one. Thus, this memory of death brings us back to what is essential, awakening another kind of attention in the here and now. This watchfulness is the pure tranquility that yoga nidra aims to make us available to. But this effort is constantly caught up by the sense of "me," by the ego and a whirlpool of thoughts that pretend to know what needs to be done, albeit wrongly; one must not be fooled by that which keeps us away from this vast peace. No matter how much effort is put in, or whatever practice or action is done, it is important to question the nature of the "me" who thinks that "I" am the author of the action and that "I" am doing it: Who is meditating? Who thinks "I" am meditating well or not meditating well? Who falls asleep? Who feels peaceful? Who dies? Who asks the question? Once all the answers of the mind are put aside, only the radiant truth, which Ramana Maharshi realized when he was seventeen years old, remains:

I was sitting alone in a room on the first floor of my uncle's house. I seldom had any sickness and on that day there was nothing wrong with my health, but a sudden violent fear of death overtook me. There was nothing in my state of health to account for it nor was there any urge in me to find out whether there was any account for the fear. I just felt I was going to die and began thinking what to do about it. It did not occur to me to consult a doctor or any elders or friends. I felt I had to solve the problem myself then and there. The shock of the fear of death drove my mind inwards and I said to myself mentally, without actually framing the words: "Now death has come; what does it mean? What is it that is dying? This body dies." And at once I dramatized the occurrence of death. I lay with my limbs stretched out still as though rigor mortis has set in, and imitated a corpse so as to give greater reality to the enquiry. I held my breath and kept my lips tightly closed so that no sound could escape, and that neither the word "I" nor any word could be uttered. "Well then," I said to myself, "this body is dead. It will be carried stiff to the burning ground and there burned and reduced to ashes. But with the death of the body, am I dead? Is the body I? It is silent and inert, but I feel the full force of my personality and even the voice of I within me, apart from it. So I am the Spirit transcending the body. The body dies but the spirit transcending it cannot be touched by death. That means I am the deathless Spirit." All this was not dull thought; it flashed through me vividly as living truths which I perceived directly almost without thought process. "I" was something real, the only real thing about my present state, and all the conscious activity connected with the body was centered on that "I." From that moment onwards, the "I" or Self focused attention on itself by a powerful fascination. Fear of death vanished once and for all. The ego was lost in the flood of Self-awareness.

Absorption in the Self continued unbroken from that time. Other thoughts might come and go like the various notes of music, but the "I" continued like the fundamental *sruti* note which underlies and blends with all other notes. Whether the body was engaged in talking, reading or anything else, I was still centered on "I." Previous to that crisis I had no perception of myself and was not consciously attracted to it. I had felt no direct perceptible interest in it, much less any permanent disposition to dwell upon it.[23]

Following this experience, the young man's life changed radically. The same opportunity is given to us every time that we practice yoga nidra with sincerity.

That being said, such cases of spontaneous awakening are rare. Even if this awakening is necessarily spontaneous, it often takes place only after years of repeated efforts. It is often when the effort ends that non-effort is understood: when the one who thinks he is the doer, exhausted by his efforts, gives up, surrenders, and fades away. Of the two, the *yogi,* motionless as a corpse, continues to walk in the meanders of the inner labyrinth and exercise this precious faculty of discrimination, to be able to differentiate the rope from the snake and the permanent from the fleeting.

Practicing yoga, just like philosophizing, is about learning how to die. According to Montaigne, "the point of all wisdom and reasoning is to teach us to no longer fear death."[24] The philosopher invites us to familiarize ourselves with it, to practice it, become accustomed to it, and keep it "in our mind" and "on our lips." "Death isn't some horrific thing, something to be avoided, something to be postponed, but rather something to be with day in and day out," Krishnamurti used to say. "And out of that comes an extraordinary sense of immensity." The Greeks would bring a corpse into the room during grand feasts. In India, some renunciants live in cremation grounds and meditate on lifeless corpses, simply using a skull as their begging bowl and for food. Montaigne also remarks that "it is as foolish to lament that we shall not be alive a hundred years from now as it is to lament that we were not alive a hundred years ago." Moreover, as Nisargadatta Maharaj would often ask, "How do we know that we did not exist a thousand years ago?" Or in Zen teachings: "What was your original face before the birth of your parents?" These questions can answer the question of death by themselves and awaken us to our true nature.

Montaigne adds that "the continual work of your life is to contrive death; you are in death during the time you continue in life . . . during life you are still 'dying.'" Thus, with yoga nidra, breath after breath, I can discover the fundamental difference between the process of death—which is inherent to every cell, every thought, and each passing moment—and the exact moment when the body will stop breathing forever. Little by little, by imitating death through conscious sleep, I can slip into the spectator's seat until my attention turns toward itself and awakens me to the indescribable splendor of Awareness. With the wiping away of "me" and "my" thoughts, the fear of death disappears along with all other fears, for it is both the keystone and the root cause of all other fears. All important spiritual traditions teach us that while we are alive, we can discover the very basis of Consciousness, and thus understand the mystery of death. To begin with, I must set aside everything I think I know about death. What remains, if I don't think about it? I am only afraid of death if I am identified with the body and thoughts, and if I do not realize that death is simply the extinction of what I think I am. The confrontation with death gives me an incredible opportunity to go beyond it; the alert perception of my finiteness makes me more aware of the peace in which life, in all its forms, dances with death itself. What I believe to be death is probably just this great silence in which I lie down every night, like a water bubble rising up in the wave, only to burst and become one with the ocean. When someone dies, it is often heard or said: "May he or she rest in peace." But the one who rests in peace is not dead. Even if what is to come is only a vague idea, this peace is already here, waiting to be recognized and inhabited, beyond everything I know or think I know:

> Krishna said: Whosoever, at the end, leaves the body,* thinking of any being, to that being only he goes . . . . Therefore, at all times, remember Me . . .[25]

---

*"Leaves the body" can also refer to when one falls asleep.

PART II

THE PRACTICE OF
YOGA NIDRA

That which is night to all beings, in that the self-controlled man keeps awake; where all beings are awake, that is the night for the Sage (Muni) who sees.

BHAGAVAD GITA, 2:69

Yoga Nidra as a Practice:
An Introduction

As you have probably noticed, the practice has already begun because the philosophy of yoga nidra never ceases to bring us back to ourselves; and this return, this remembering of the Self and coming back to oneself is the heart of yoga nidra. Although the path of conscious sleep is different and independent by itself, it can easily be adapted to all other practices of presence and adopted by all people, allowing one to experience the practices deeply and in a different way, with a new quality of relaxation and renewed attention.

In concrete terms, yoga nidra will first teach us how to cultivate relaxation as a means for becoming more available to awareness in sleep, dreams, and wakefulness, and also as a prerequisite to every practice. I must first learn how to detect and undo tensions and tightness, by differentiating the tensions of the physical, energetic, and mental areas, even though they are all linked with one another. And this in itself is a vast program that calls for alert observation. It is necessary to distinguish the preparatory techniques and the reminder techniques, which allow one to approach sleep and the presence to oneself in general, from the practice sessions per se. We must try to recognize what the human being is, as a species (in evolution), as a part of nature and the universe, in its profound essence and according to the laws that dictate phenomena. It is also necessary to differentiate the practices to be done during the day from those to be done in bed, when one falls asleep or when one wakes up during the night, and when one wakes up in the morning. Yoga nidra can also be used in therapy. In a general manner, a symbol can become a means to link together levels that coexist, but that do not necessarily communicate with one another. For example, the symbolic process of energy centers is used to orient the mind and attune it with its energetic reality, even if the symbol is evidently not the center itself. Yoga nidra deals with important, fundamental themes related to human beings such as desire, fear, animality, time, love, death, or sexual ecstasy by inviting us to constantly renew our conscious vision of the structures that constitute us, such as the senses, the body, the wheels of energy, the meridians, the mental processes, and so forth. Regardless of how we look at it, yoga nidra always bring us back to the essence, which can only exist in silence, in the void, joy, and quietude of the heart, and in the unique taste of pure presence without object.

This is why, more than phenomena, yoga nidra will invite us to observe the intervals, the spaces, and the transition from one posture to another, from one breath to another, and from one state to another. This is why we play with modifications, reversal, points of view, falling asleep, waking up, and pauses or intervals. In this way, yoga nidra teaches us to observe the mind's processes, and how the mind goes from awareness to unawareness, from sleep to the dream state, and so on, even though the states are not really separated from one another. I am awake, but still I dream; I am dreaming, but still I am awake. It is all mixed up. Yoga nidra will help us to understand and know how the mind that is required to survive in this world functions, because I cannot live in harmony with others if I do not understand what is happening at the thought level. The practice will thus allow us to differentiate the mind (just an organ among others that is simply considered to be the sixth sense) from Awareness and from the Self. If I do not understand this difference, I will never understand myself and I will always be controlled by the mind. It is just an organ with life in it, just like a light bulb with electricity. By observing the pauses or intervals, by playing with the transition from one point of view to another and by exploring the intervals, I may be able to recognize the intervals' true nature. Irrespective of whether it is between balance and imbalance, between two thoughts, two postures, two experiences, or two states, the space that connects them is always the same, for it is the very substratum in which everything takes place. A few years ago, my face looked young, now it looks old. The one who thinks it is "my" face never used to pay much attention to it earlier, where as now, "I" am worried about it. But the vision that is aware of all this never changes. It is the awareness in which everything appears and passes on. This type of practice, aiming to explore the structures of the being, is obviously linked with the deep experiences that the practitioner desires to have or renew in his or her imagination. The attention focused on the interval does not seek to enjoy an experience, but only to recognize the background in which all experiences happen; they happen, but the background remains ever peaceful, free from the phenomena that appear and disappear in it. This is at the heart of yoga nidra and this reality is evoked by Nisargadatta Maharaj in the following passage:

Question: Sir, of what use to me is your telling me that reality cannot be found in consciousness? Where else am I to look for it? How do you apprehend it?

Maharaj: It is quite simple. If I ask you what is the taste of your mouth all you can do is to say: it is neither sweet nor bitter, nor sour nor astringent; it is what remains when all these tastes are not. Similarly, when all distinctions and reactions are no more, what remains is reality, simple and solid.[1]

In addition to this immersion into the source of all things, yoga nidra also allows us to explore archetypes of species and myths. The state of wakefulness imprisons and restricts, but in sleep one can explore archetypes and symbols related to all species and the universe. Yoga nidra makes it possible to go deep into each structure that composes us, starting from the gross and the most dense matter and going into the more subtle and vibrant matter; it allows us to go beyond the small ego and open up to that which surpasses it. Yoga nidra is a journey that observes how the machine works, overviewing all species, the universe, the microcosmos and the macrocosmos, the individual and the absolute, in deep observation of the appearing of every phenomenon, until the race ends in the observer. It is truly a journey into the states of matter, consciousness, and joy of being. From there should emerge a feeling of balance, peace, harmony, and joy that goes beyond the simple prospect of being aware in each state, extending to every moment of our daily life. By contemplating the river of life flowing by, without getting carried away by its strong current, the word *contentment* will take on a whole new meaning, joy will have a whole new flavor, and life will have a whole new radiance, revealing the river and all its beauty.

These practices will guide us to these states of awareness, allow us to court them, to come and go from one state to another. Contrary to common belief, in our case "a good night's sleep" is when I wake up during the night and know that I am sleeping peacefully; I reach a state of still awareness and am a witness to the body and thoughts that are asleep. If everything seems more orderly in the state of wakefulness, the habitual order of the mind disappears when I am asleep. It loses the layout of its waking state, allowing me to break through the barriers that habitually operate. When I am asleep, everything falls away and there are no limits; and this is when a marvelous journey can begin. The structure of the mind becomes a labyrinth in which I can navigate in a different manner. I can go into the depths of myself, discover what I am not, and allow what I am to reveal itself. This kind of practice can result in the capacity to sleep less, to feel rested with less sleep in a short time, not to mention the fact that we will not waste one third of our lives sleeping. Thus, it is important to accept and savor the moments of clarity, in lighter and more luminous sleep; it is important to relax, abandon oneself, and efface oneself completely. What I truly am will reveal itself on its own, independently, beyond what I can see and the idea I have of what it is, or beyond any sense of progression. This is why it is necessary to be disciplined, humble, and nonchalant in this practice, accomplishing it without desire for results and attachment to the act. Simply and peacefully, only for relishing the presence to oneself.

The Limbs of Yoga According to the Nidra Tradition

In yoga nidra, we will rediscover the eight limbs or steps of traditional yoga, in their classical as well as adapted versions: poses, breathing exercises, locks, gestures, concentrations, recital of sacred verses, and so on. Each step is an opportunity to stop the fluctuations of the mind, to be in meditation and in complete awareness, regardless of whether it is done in a sitting posture, lying down, or while moving. The main characteristic of yoga nidra is that it insists on the zones of transition, like when we fall asleep, in the natural pausing of thoughts, and at the same time remaining perfectly alert. "The dispersive activity of the mind creates a kind of eddy, and while it stirs, the vast peace of the Ocean beyond cannot be felt,"[2] yogi Sri Anirvan explains. This is why it is necessary to remain "alert and aware," and it is possible "to use the natural absence of the mind's activity to serve the goal of yoga," whether this absence is due to sleeping, sneezing, having an orgasm, fainting, or any other ordinary "loss of consciousness." "Just as I am alert and aware when the vibration of the mind's activity carries on vigorously," Sri Anirvan adds, "I must strive to remain in that way when it slows down or stops altogether":

> Sleep is to remain in the state of samadhi—this is the formula for yogic practice. In meditation we forcibly try to stop the activity of the mind, but in sleep this stoppage occurs by itself, but because I cannot yet transform my sleep, my mind sinks into oblivion or gets excited by unwanted distractions. Yet the very aim of sleep is to find peace and to refresh and energize the mind by returning to the Origin, the Cause (*mahakarana*). The Origin is the Mother, She who, in the language of the Upanishads, is the Ruler of All (*sarveshvari*), the Womb of All (*sarvayoni*), and the Enjoyer of Bliss

(*anadabhuk*). Sleep is the invocation of this very Mother. It is also a Yoga, and with a bit of technique all the limbs of Yoga can be applied.[3]

POSES

The poses (asana), in their classical versions, will first let the body relax and attune with the breathing and thought processes, thus awakening a new quality of presence to oneself. They should not be executed like a performance or in a spirit of competition, but in total awareness, with alert attention and without expecting any results, as if each time is the first time. We do this by focusing our attention on gravity and on the bodily sensations, on every breath and on the vibrations that appear and disappear; by taking the pose gracefully and relishing this presence to the movements of the body and the mind. The posture allows me to see how I am and where I am at each moment, and how I am in life, with my desires and aversions. Each pose offers a different observation of oneself, contrary to the limited poses that I adopt in my daily life, at the office or sprawled out on the couch. The pose familiarizes me with what I am not. It becomes the basis for extensive listening and a preview to the feeling of profound tranquility. In order to experience this, it is necessary to open up to the vibratory dimension of the body and to the space in which the pose is taken and undone. The pose can awaken me to the space in the body, between each joint. I visualize the pose before I do it, according to the flexibility of the structures of the mind and energy. I allow the pose to take place, without imposing it or forcing it in any way; the pose is like opening up, being available, exploring, listening, and tasting. There is nothing to master and nothing to obtain or attain; just alert and equanimous listening of the contractions, sensations, and empty spaces in the body. There is neither desire nor aversion. Let the conditioning undo itself, without creating a new one. Open up to the spontaneity of the moment, to the sensitivity, to the free expansion of forms and the alphabet of the postures. Be an alert and silent witness, listening to the phenomenon. Pose after pose, I allow my attention to let go and awaken to its true substance. "The only true posture that counts," Ramana Maharshi used to say, "is to stay in the Self." This pose, formless and effortless, does not substitute others, but can be added to them all; the other poses appear and disappear in this pose. It is not an action, but an impersonal witness of the action. As a result, nobody does it; but it simply is.

The alphabet of the poses can also be an answer to some elementary grammatical rules that are operative as well as symbolic, in order to form words, small phrases, and actual poetry, composed or improvised, in the spontaneity of the moment, without knowing what will appear from one moment to the next. For example, it is possible to practice the poses in the ascending order of the energy centers, like we do with the focusing of attention in yoga nidra sessions. This kind of rule is in relation to the inherent logic of the withdrawal of the senses, to the process of the effacement of "me," and to the resorption of the gross and subtle elements. Each pose can potentially be paired up with specific breathing and concentration, but always in the intimate conjugation of relaxation and attention.

After a purification exercise like the classical sun salutation, a powerful energy comes into the body, warming it up, thus regenerating and prepping it to start its day and to do other poses.[4] Among the eighty-four postures mentioned in the texts, some can be adapted to yoga nidra. For example:

- the standing posture
- tree pose
- triangle pose
- palms and hands to the feet
- lotus pose
- mountain pose
- intense west stretch pose
- cobra pose

- locust pose
- bow pose
- crocodile pose
- boat pose
- twisting pose
- diamond pose (seated and lying down)
- child's pose
- balance pose
- fish pose
- crow pose
- cat pose
- cow face pose
- half fish pose
- eight limb pose
- plough pose
- wheel pose
- all prayer postures
- all postures that open the heart center (which is in direct relation with the sense of touch and sleep)
- headstand
- corpse pose

These last two are especially effective for their stillness, which offers infinite possibilities for yoga nidra on two different levels of practice.

"First, lie down in the dead-body posture (*shavasana*), absolutely motionless. Then, through relaxation, spread out the body-consciousness like a rarefied gas. This is *asana*."[5]

BREATHING

Once the physical pose is taken, I can simply observe the natural rise and fall of my breathing, without trying to control it. I can also do a specific breathing exercise (*pranayama*). For example, inhale one beat, exhale two beats (1:2); or inhale one beat, hold for four beats and exhale two beats (1:4:2); or in the same way, but keeping the lungs empty, which would signify inhale four seconds, exhale eight seconds, and sixteen seconds of breath suspension. Numerous breathing exercises exist in classical hatha yoga that can be perfectly adapted to yoga nidra, such as even breathing, uneven breathing, four-part breathing, breathing to purify the channels, breath of the victorious or conquering, the bee breath, and the breath of blackout (of the mind).

"Next, pay attention to the breathing for awhile, making it full and rhythmic. Then, in consonance with the breathing, do japa by continuously repeating the seed *mantra* Hamsa, saying Ham while breathing out, Sa while breathing in. This is *pranayama*."[6]

It is more about listening to the natural mantra repeating itself through us, than actually saying it. I simply observe my breathing. I welcome its rise and fall; I allow it to stretch out like waves on the infinite horizon. My breath draws out, my body and thoughts relax, let go, and come undone. A benevolent space begins to open up. The meaning of the mantra is revealed: "I am."

GESTURES AND LOCKS

The gestures and locks in yoga (*mudra* and *bandha*) can also be practiced independently or combined with postures and breathing exercises. Among the most important are the root lock, the abdominal lock, and the neck lock. Eye movements and focused gazes also occupy an important place, all the more so because they are closely linked with the fire centers, with the toes and thumbs, the stomach, the whole spine, with the circulation of energy, and with dreams. The contractions of the sphincter and the perineum, as well as the tongue locks and hand gestures, also occupy an important place in this subtle and sensorial mechanism. The gesture of the ears, particularly of interest in yoga nidra, can directly activate the vital breath that controls the act of yawning. The technique is simple: pinch your ear lobes with your thumb and index finger, pull them down as much as possible, and simultaneously, open your mouth and stick out your tongue, making sure it touches no part of your mouth, with its tip pointing slightly backward, open your eyes wide, lift up your eyebrows as high as possible . . . And that should get you to yawn. This is a beautiful gesture of relaxation and energy, something to do before a yoga nidra session, before you fall asleep or when you wake up, or whenever you like. It can be done simply for the pleasure of feeling at peace.

WITHDRAWAL OF THE SENSES AND CONCENTRATION

After the poses, gestures, and breathing exercises have awakened a more subtle sensitivity of the body and its vibrations—and created a context suitable for introspection—the attention can begin to go deeper into the inner layers. It is necessary to gradually be free from the hold of the senses, just like before we fall asleep. In order to do this, I can become aware of the sense of smell, then of taste, of sight, of touch, and of hearing, one by one, in relation to the corresponding energy centers. First, I become aware of faraway sounds, and then gradually, I bring my attention to sounds in my place of practice, until I hear the sound of silence itself. I can also focus on an inspiring image or a beam of light behind my eyes, allowing it to become smaller and smaller until it becomes a minuscule dot disappearing into the formless and colorless. I can also sense a part of the body, like the spine, and allow the subtle touch of the vibrant feeling to lead me to an even deeper stillness. This withdrawal of the senses will thus allow for better concentration on an inner, more subtle support, such as a specific energy center or flow. The play of the limbs of yoga seeks only to suspend thoughts and open us to the unknown by connecting alert watchfulness with deep relaxation and tranquility.

At the same time picture yourself in the image of Narayana lying in eternal repose, and let the resulting mood spread in yourself.

It is not upon your bed that you lie, but upon the infinite Causal Ocean of light. Upon this ocean your spinal column floats and it is charged with electricity. Now draw your whole consciousness into your heart; from there imagine your consciousness coursing upward, in an ineffable stream of sensation, to the throat center, the forehead center, and then through the crown of the head into the Void. Above, below, to the right and left there is only the vast emptiness of an unsupported infinite Sky. From it the Mother, in the form of Yoga-sleep, descends into your heart and then again flows heavenward into the consciousness above the head. This is *pratyahara* and *dharana*. By practicing this, it is possible to transform your sleep.[7]

MEDITATION AND DEEP CONTEMPLATION

Now we come to a point where it is impossible to "do" anything more. When I truly recognize that the void of the heart and the void of the fontanel are one, the thought or feeling of being a separate entity disappears completely. Thus, only pure awareness remains, totally impersonal and tranquil, without a subject who is seeing and without an object that is seen, like an original vision, an uncreated vision. Even the slightest intention of doing something or becoming something will ruin everything. "I" am not meditating, and it is only by realizing this that the illusion can disappear and allow the peace of the void to emerge; this is true meditation. Meditation does not belong to the field of doing something. Meditation is not an action. This is the understanding that yoga nidra brings to us. It is *dhyana* and *samadhi*.

Preparatory Exercises

The art of yoga nidra consists in uniting the limbs of yoga to serve its goal. Some specific exercises can be done independently and constitute an excellent preparation for conscious sleep and also for longer yoga nidra sessions.

Simply lying down in the corpse pose and staying perfectly still, without doing anything, is in itself a marvelous exercise. And certainly the most difficult one. It is both the alpha and the omega, the union of the first and last letter of the Sanskrit alphabet (*a-ham,* I Am). It is the exercise I start with, and to which all the limbs of yoga bring me back. Simply, lying down, "being," without words or thoughts.

Lying down on the ground, arms and legs slightly apart, palms facing upward and the back firmly placed on the floor: this is the basic pose in all formal yoga nidra sessions. It is with this pose that one gently slips into the stillness of sleep and of death. It is possible to adjust the pose with a cushion under one's head or knees so as to avoid contractions in the lumber region. To each his own, be it in life, in death, or in the corpse pose. I make sure to let go of my body, particularly of my face, hands, arms, shoulders, neck, my whole back, and my legs, aware of their contact with the floor. I become aware of the air entering the nostrils, warmer as it comes out, inhaling and exhaling, giving and taking, living and dying. Breath after breath, I give way to the stillness and inertia, to the tranquil background, a witness to that which appears and disappears. I become fixed in the unchanging and in the awareness. The breath becomes thin and subtle, almost nonexistent, like a corpse that is no longer breathing. Like in tantric yoga, I relish this still peace, taking pleasure in being, simply being, until I forget and no longer know that I am. Contradictions and duality then dissolve in immense peace.

> *Then even nothingness was not, nor existence,*
> *There was no air then, nor the heavens beyond it.*
> *What covered it? Where was it? In whose keeping*
> *Was there then cosmic water, in depths unfathomed?*
>
> *Then there was neither death nor immortality*
> *Nor was there then the torch of night and day.*

The One breathed windlessly and self-sustaining.
There was that One then, and there was no other.

At first there was only darkness wrapped in darkness.
All this was only unillumined water.
That One which came to be, enclosed in nothing,
arose at last, born of the power of heat.

In the beginning desire descended on it.
That was the primal seed, born of the mind.
The sages who have searched their hearts with wisdom
know that which is kin to that which is not.

And they have stretched their cord across the void,
And know what was above, and what below.
Seminal powers made fertile mighty forces.
Below was strength, and over it was impulse.

But, after all, who knows, and who can say
Whence it all came, and how creation happened?
The gods themselves are later than creation,
So who knows truly whence it has arisen?

Whence all creation had its origin,
He, whether he fashioned it or whether he did not,
He, who surveys it all from highest heaven,
He knows—or maybe even he does not know.[8]

Still lying down on my back, I inhale and take my arms overhead until the backs of my hands touch the floor; at this moment, the breath stops, and during this retention of breath I clasp my hands and arch my body, becoming aware of my whole body and the vibrant space around it, before bringing my arms back to my sides while exhaling. The exercise can be repeated several times, focusing more and more on the retention of the breath: I can do it once, with the sensation of the physical body, once in the energetic structure (or in the energy centers one by one), and once in the infinite space of the mind. At the end of this exercise, I take a minute to relish and feel the stillness of being.

In addition to the corpse pose, I can also consciously relax and seek stillness in the tree pose or the headstand.

For the tree pose, stand straight, with your feet firmly placed on the ground, then place one ankle on the inner side your thigh, close to the perineum, and balance on one leg. Place your arms on each side, slightly away from the body, in the gesture of wisdom or the palms joined in front of the chest, in the prayer gesture. I stay like this, allow the tensions to come undone and the breath to calm down, with a gaze of attention and tranquility.

Exercises for Falling Asleep

Among all yoga practices, those that consist in observing the process of falling asleep are the most indispensable and by far the most important, not only at night, but also before naps, long practice sessions, and short preparatory exercises.

In the practice of yoga nidra, it is necessary to know one's "sleeper's breathing." In the beginning, you can sit back against a cushion with your legs stretched out, or simply lie down comfortably on your back or in the position in which you fall asleep easily and naturally. You can practice in your bed, as the aim is to fall asleep quickly and wake up several times, in order to observe the breathing process and observe your "sleeper's breathing." Once it is learned, I can respond to it in order to fall asleep on command or as quickly as possible, and thus begin a deeper practice. Naps become a wonderful time for practicing. In the beginning, if I do not totally understand how this process works, I can imitate the common way to do it, based on my own observations.

The breath rises with each inhalation, stretches a little, then falls down with each exhalation and dissolves in a short pause with the lungs empty. By deliberately imitating this rhythm, my own sleeper's breathing sets in rapidly and spontaneously. There is nothing to do, and I must certainly not interfere in the process in order to be able to see it as it is and not as I believe it to be. In this practice, I am happy observing the phenomenon at work. Listening is centered on the air entering and coming out of the nostrils (or of the more active nostril, if possible) and on the sense of touch. I allow my breath to become like the sleeper's breathing; I imitate it and let it happen. A few minutes before I fall asleep, the breathing changes, and each breath becomes longer, stretches out, and pauses in the natural retention of the empty lungs. The breath slowly dwindles. The body falls asleep and consumes less oxygen. I do not try to resist, but I let myself go. Images and sounds appear faster and faster. Everything loses it consistency. The breath keeps changing: rising and falling, empty pauses, the interval, sleep . . . Conscious or unconscious? What does the interval taste like? If I cannot be conscious when I fall asleep, what will happen when I die?

Once I am familiarized with this sleeper's breathing, it is possible to fall asleep in classical hatha yoga postures, which I can eventually adjust for this practice, maybe by choosing more simple and comfortable postures. For example, the tortoise pose, diamond pose, or child's pose are three postures that stimulate the energy center of sleep. Thus, they are perfect for this practice. The pose should be comfortable; otherwise it is impossible to fall asleep. The aim is to study the process that precedes the act of falling asleep and to play with the transition from one state to the other. For example, the diamond pose consists in sitting with the buttocks on the heels, arms alongside the body. And child's pose begins here and consists of then leaning forward until the chest is on the thighs and the forehead is touching the floor or placed on a cushion. In both poses, I can relax and slowly slip into the sleeper's breathing.

No matter which posture or support I use, the sequence is always the same: I establish slow and light breathing (possibly by synchronizing it with one or several sacred words); the gaze is centered and conscious of the infinite space behind the eyes. I greet the first signs of falling asleep: the physiological, respiratory, and mental modifications.

Physiologically speaking, the body and its tensions are completely undone, a state of relaxation is established, the senses are interiorized and break down, and the body temperature drops. This link with the cold is important in yoga nidra because it keeps one slightly awake, as opposed to heat, which brings heaviness. The cold connects us with the tactile feeling, with the sense of touch and the skin, and hence, in accordance with the interdependent elements, with the heart center or the center of sleep. This is why during the practice of yoga nidra I should try to leave my body as uncovered as possible, in order to feel the cold and get used to the feeling of coolness. This feeling is a sign that I am about to fall asleep; but moreover, it allows me to wake up again and connect with the heart center. On the skin, this coolness is felt at the time of falling asleep, like the skin of something empty and, like a "bag of skin," empty of physiological content. Thus, the coolness felt on the skin helps by guiding me in my practice. Furthermore, to feel well in one's skin means to feel it in the first place. If necessary, one must not hesitate to cover oneself.

As for the modifications of the mind, its order and consistency disappear. While falling asleep, the mind is deconstructed, it loses its structure of the waking state and the thoughts come undone. I penetrate into a different world with the impression that I am entering and burying myself in a deep corridor, with images or flashes that flow faster and faster as sleep approaches. The dormant impressions are seen under a new gaze. If I perceive the thought associations in relation to the day's events, I can see more images surfacing spontaneously at the threshold of sleep—images that are related to the past, but are still identifiable—as well as other unknown images that I recognize without being able to connect them with any known source.

As far as the respiratory modifications are concerned, when sleep approaches the breath and the sleeper's breathing become one. If I am lying down on my right side, in the position of the reclining Buddha, I focus my attention on the left nostril, simultaneously listening to the inner sound, until I consciously and peacefully slip into the sleep state. I try to fall asleep while maintaining the subtle sensation of breath and sound at the same time, and I try to find it again immediately after waking up, as if both states were connected by the sensation of a very subtle and almost imperceptible vibration appearing like a golden thread, a precious guide in the meanders of the different states of consciousness. In this way I can truly understand the interconnection between sleep and breath, as well as the sharpness of attention required to observe it.

> One should concentrate on the state when sleep has not yet come, but the external awareness has disappeared (between waking and sleep)—there the supreme Goddess reveals herself.[9]

The act of falling asleep is composed of the short preparatory phase followed by the phase of emptiness, where ordinary consciousness fades away into sleep. This setting is the space that opens up to a void full of light, like the pale reflection of the moon. Another way to do this is to lie down in corpse pose, where I can let the breath stretch out and become as long as possible without using too much air. I observe this and let the sounds and images flow. I am a spectator, fading away in the pause after exhaling, in the heart center. I go to the other side of the mirror. I fall asleep and wake up, relishing the rise and fall of my breathing and its caress that leads me to that which creates and to this Life.

Other methods also exist to make the holding of attention easier when one falls asleep, like falling asleep and waking up with the inner sound and the active nostril. This exercise connects air and space with the heart and throat centers, and to the senses of touch and hearing. By allowing me to remain alert up to the point where the senses are completely broken down, this exercise carries me to the threshold of sleep. If I am lying down on my right side, the air will naturally flow more through my left nostril and the sound will be more perceptible in my left ear, thus activating the lunar aspect. It is the opposite if I am lying down on my left side. On my back, the perception is more subtle, as the breathing is balanced and the sound is more noticeable. Thus I bring my attention to my breathing and observe in which nostril the breath flows more freely. I remain concentrated on that nostril and on the active side, and then I slowly start my sleeper's breathing. I then allow my attention to extend to the sound of my deep and peaceful breathing. I am aware of everything that is happening, to all phenomena that appear in my consciousness and to the pause after exhalation, in order to greet the moment when sleep approaches. Here, the idea is to fall asleep while being alert until the very last minute, with my attention on my breathing, inextricably linked to its subtle feeling or to its sound—or to both—in order to remember one or both as soon as I wake up. The aim is to recognize the connection between both states of consciousness.

> How can one preserve this alive sensation of oneself in sleep? The first effort is to try and enter sleep consciously by remaining in a very subtle sensation of oneself that will continue far beyond the state of ordinary consciousness falling into the heaviness of sleep, and become one with a vibration of life whose process is absolutely known. When one wakes up, the reverse happens. This vibration will unfold to animate the sensation of oneself, long before the body wakes up.[10]

The link between these two states cannot be created or produced. It can only be recognized. However, to become aware of the energy centers, elements, senses, and their close connection, one must be totally open and available. This is why training oneself to fall asleep in yoga postures that connect us with the heart center, thereby connecting us with the sense of touch and sleep, allows us to understand those physiological and energetic interconnections. I can thus take the tortoise pose or child's pose, by observing my breath, its vibration, and its sound, and move into the fetal position just as I am about to fall asleep. Slowly but surely in this way I can learn how to fall asleep superficially or more deeply, all the while maintaining a certain kind of attention. The process of falling asleep appears with more clarity and I can thus divide it into different phases, following the order of the breakdown of the senses and associating each one of them with, for example, a bright circle of a particular color and intensity. I am thus able to recognize this clear light, like the moon adorning Shiva's forehead. This clear light is no longer a perceived object, like a circle of color, but the Consciousness itself in which the "I" goes from wakefulness to sleep. Sri Ramakrishna, as well as tantric texts, advise us that it is important to commit ourselves to "voluntary sleep coming from the heart and not from an inferior center." I can train myself by bringing the attention in the heart center, on a bright circle or point as mentioned earlier, or on the continuous unbeaten inner sound (*anahata shabda*), by trying to fall asleep in the empty pauses, in order to become aware of the important interval.

> With a little effort this moment can be prolonged. At the time of sleep, the mind naturally tends toward cessation of activity; this tendency can be cultivated so that it comes very slowly, feeling its way. One should not snuff out the lamp all at once, but sink into sleep as the daylight vanishes into the bosom of the evening, as the child falls asleep on the breast of its mother. No, this last simile is not yet complete. The child falls asleep, but the mother remains awake. The child may have a sort of trust that his mother stays awake, but he is not very aware of it. In yogic sleep (*yoganidra*), that awareness will be pronounced and clear.[11]

If all efforts seem to fail, you must certainly not feel frustration or despair. Allow the comments and judgments to pass, and continue your practice; remain in the present moment without tormenting yourself. Feeling pride or feeling self-pity is the same thing, and it only reinforces the ego and the sense of "me" who thinks that she is the author of her actions, and consequently, of her practices. And this only leads to a dead end. I must on the contrary surrender, give in, fade away, open up, and let myself go in the rapture, like Saint Teresa of Ávila, as described by Fray Francisco de Osuna in this inspiring and inspired text:

> Blessed are those who practice contemplative prayer before they sleep and those who promptly go back to it when they wake up. They eat a little, sleep, eat a little more and nestle in the Lord's arms, like children who fall asleep on their mother's breast after being fed, then they wake up, suckle some more and fall asleep again. Thus, in these radiant intervals, their time is spent more in contemplative prayer than in sleep . . . even though they have slept; when they wake up they know that their soul has slept in the Beloved's arms.[12]

Yogi Sri Anirvan awakens the same feeling of total abandon when he talks of the Mother, that is the Consciousness, this "limpid clearness as of pale moonlight":

> The whole of our day is busily spent on work. We say to our Mother: "O Mother, we have no time to invoke you. Where is the time to sit awhile and call you? This is why we do not remember you." But the Mother does not forget us. In the depths of every night She extinguishes our world of busy work and clamorous thought. In her deep compassion, she draws us into the fathomless depths of her Yoga-heart, into the pristine river of knowledge flowing back to its source. Even if I do not know, the Mother knows. Even if I can give her nothing else, if only I could give her my sleep. If only I could tell her, "In lying down, I lie at your feet; in sleeping I think only of you."[13]

Exercises for the Night

Yoga nidra can also be practiced during sleeplessness and when we wake up during the night, either deliberately or spontaneously. Normally, when I am in an ordinary state of consciousness, the cycle begins with a slow and light sleep during which I am very sensitive to the noise outside. In slow and deep sleep, the body is completely at rest and I hear nothing. Brain activity begins once again with paradoxical sleep or the dream state. This activity of the mind is manifested by an increase in brain waves and rapid eye movements. After a latent period, the body wakes up or starts a new cycle of approximately one and a half hours. Four cycles correspond approximately to a six-hour night, naturally offering numerous intervals that we can explore.

> (. . .) night time, with its silence, should first be dedicated to the gradual work of conscious interiorization, then to voluntary sleep in a state of awakened consciousness. This sleep in a body without fatigue or tension (except the minimal wear and tear caused by time) and in a practiced pose, that never changes, becomes the field for numerous experiments.[14]

Practices that consist in setting an alarm several times during the night as an intentional wake-up call should not be carried out without the guidance of a very able teacher, and only for short periods of time and in very favorable conditions; otherwise they will only bring fatigue and confusion. This is why it is preferable to use the moments when we wake up naturally and spontaneously during the night to come back to a session that began at the time of falling asleep, for example. Or, more simply, when I wake up spontaneously, I can immediately do a classic yoga nidra posture, such as the corpse pose, lying on my back, or Buddha's pose, lying on my right side. The pose must be done effortlessly and without agitation so that I can continue to relish the interval. I stay in the heart center, observe my breathing, and fall back asleep. When I wake up, I can also simply turn my body, stretch out, observe a dot of light, or start a breathing exercise. As always, it is important to remain tranquil and alert, and to surrender to the blessed vacuity:

> Sleep is like the Yoga-heart of the Mother. In the depths of the nights, the Earth lies asleep, but meanwhile the Sky (*akasha*) stays awake and looks on through the unblinking gaze of myriads of stars. The Sky is truly the heart of the Mother. To be asleep there means to be awake to the vast peace of the Sky. This awakening takes place very slowly, just as the moon rises slowly, diluting the darkness of evening with its spreading white light. The sleep of Yoga is like that.[15]

Exercises for Waking Up

The morning alarm, like all moments when I wake up, is as important as the moment when I fall asleep. It allows me to observe the process in reverse. Be it at dawn or dusk, the interval always offers the same possibility: to recognize one's true nature. Just as the sense of "me" disappears gradually when I fall asleep, it resurfaces every time I wake up. The moment when the sense of "I" resurfaces is a perfect opportunity to witness the resurgence of the sensory and material world, with its share of desire, aversion, and suffering. It is an opportunity to realize that this sense of "me" is only an idea that emerges when I am identified with the body.*

---

*Every time I wake up, I can perform a "rotation of consciousness" (described in the second and third parts of the book), and come out of bed with a sensation of the whole body, before pursuing my activities with presence.

There is a story about Janaka, the famous Indian king, who woke up one morning feeling a little disturbed; he had dreamed that he was just a menial laborer. So he wondered if it was King Janaka who had just dreamed that he was a laborer, or if he was a laborer dreaming that he was King Janaka. The question is certainly disturbing, but once again it appears only with the identification to a conditioned form, be it in a dream or in wakefulness. Whether I think I am King Janaka or a laborer, Chuang-tzu or a butterfly, I remain the painful toy of thoughts. Peace comes only when I realize that I am neither of them. And this calls for being present to the first thought that arises when the dream appears.

Yoga of Dreams—Svapna Yoga

The best way to be conscious of one's dreams at night is to become conscious of one's dreams during the day. In wakefulness, I spend most of my time daydreaming, lost in my thoughts. If I am not aware of this *now,* then I can never be aware of it during nocturnal dreams. That being said, tantric yoga mentions practices that bring about total awareness in the dream state. Contrary to lucid dreaming, yoga nidra or svapna yoga, does not aim at mastering or realizing one's dreams, and consequently reinforcing the sense of "me" and its basic desires. Yoga nidra simply invites me to be aware that I am dreaming when I am dreaming. This in itself is more than enough.

Svapna yoga offers practices that can be explored like a game, with the mindset of a child who sees the world for the very first time. For example, in the state of wakefulness, it is possible to do an exercise that consists in the elaboration of a scenario implying the five senses, and extracting the image that resumes it in the best way from it. Then, by remembering this image in the moments of interval, like when one falls asleep, sneezes, or has an orgasm, or during particular breathing exercises, eye movements, and other exercises related to the fire element where a specific amount of energy is available, the impression that remains will be even more forceful and likely to emerge in dreams. If this has also been practiced during sessions, the resurgence of the sensory image in dreams will allow one to be aware of it, awakening to the dream, without waking up. One can then experience a moment of awareness that is luminous and extremely agreeable.

Let us note the importance of the energy center of the navel area—particularly active during the dream state—and remember the connection that this region maintains with the fire element, with the sense of vision, the big toes, the anus, and the whole central channel. One can easily note that visual impressions are the most remarkable and they are imprinted more rapidly on the mind, thus occupying an important place in our dreams and in our memory. This is why, in the case of dream yoga, it is naturally easier to work with an image rather than with a scent, even though this may vary from person to person. The sense of touch is also important and this is why yoga nidra stresses the importance of sensations and the inner feeling of the body and energy structure. For an impression to surface, the contact between a sense organ and a sensory object (internal or external) is necessary. And if I am attentive and present to myself and to the world when I receive an impression, I can feel its vibration in the energy centers and in the physical body, for example, in the central channel and in the solar plexus. The vibration in the solar plexus often indicates the rising of an emotion or the reaction of the body to the mind, but sometimes it also indicates the awakening to another mode of understanding. Observing the processes of memory and dreams can also be done by working on the other centers and through other essential themes, for example: love, possession, fear, pleasure, loss, meetings, and, last but not least, death—the secret path that guides the yoga nidra practitioner toward peace of the soul and clarity of the mind. Here there is a vast field of investigation only waiting to be explored.

With or without an image, and no matter what breathing is

operating, tantric teachings always invite us to fall asleep in the heart center. If the breath's energy is meditated upon as gross and feeble in the heart space and in the space above the fontanel, and entering the heart (at the time of sleeping), then one will attain mastery over one's dreams.[16] Yoga nidra considers the heart to be a space of initiation, the very center in which the transition toward sleep is organized. When I am about to fall asleep, all the content of my personal history and sensory experiences disappears into that space. This allows me to set intuition free and grasp my mental and emotional content, the dormant tendencies that compose my personality and behavior, in the sense that this content is not limited by the order and intelligence of my waking state. Thus the door to the conditioning of my waking and dream states is unlocked, making me more available to a preview of the Unconditioned. In Vedanta or tantric traditions, the heart, in addition to being an organ and an energy center, designates the fourth state itself, the state of yoga nidra, the nondual awareness, the Being, bliss without object, vacuity, and the Self, in which everything appears and disappears.

Which is the self? This infinite entity (*purusha*) that is identified with the intellect and is in the midst of the organs, the self-effulgent light within the heart.

Now there is this city of Brahman (the body), and in it the place, the small lotus (the heart) and in it that small ether (*Akasha*). Now what exists within that small ether is to be sought, that is to be understood.

He who knows Brahman attains the supreme goal. Brahman is the abiding reality, he is pure knowledge, and he is infinity. He who knows that Brahman dwells within the lotus of the heart, becomes one with him and enjoys all blessings[17]

Protocol for Yoga Nidra

ORGANIZING AND CREATING PRACTICE SESSIONS FOR ONESELF OR FOR OTHERS

The way in which a yoga nidra session is conducted depends on the school. In the 1940s, Swami Satyananda developed some aspects of this technique and created a systematic method, which he started teaching at the beginning of the 1960s; twenty years later, his first books were published.[18] He has, in a certain way, popularized yoga nidra. But this practical philosophy, whose source is lost in the dawn of time, of Vishnu and Shiva, cannot be reduced to just one way of being taught and practiced, and not even to a thousand ways. It all depends on the teachings that one has received, on the influences and sensitivity of the person, and how he adapts the method to himself. Yoga nidra, like all authentic traditions, continuously reminds us to open up, pause the mind, and surrender. Therefore, it would be a real shame to give too much importance to the finger pointing to the moon while forgetting to look at the moon itself, which appears in the sky of consciousness.

Like all phenomena, a typical practice session has a beginning, middle, and an end, and there are many ways to start and end a session. That being said, repeating an exercise helps a lot to relax and let go, especially in the beginning, because when one knows what one is holding on to, it is easier to let go of it. But one must also make sure that it does not become a mechanical action, and if a new exercise is chosen, one must make sure not to be caught up in the mind. Yoga nidra always calls for being on one's guard yet free from tension.

Ideally, after a classical hatha yoga session, with its poses, breathing exercises, and gestures, the session can be organized into six to ten phases, and it all depends on how one counts or divides the sequence. What is important is the consistency in the conjugation of the limbs of yoga. A general practice session has been described here, which can be adapted according to one's needs, repeating the exercises that have been practiced before. On this basis, it is possible to compose thousands of sessions for visiting the interval. In any case, the Self alone is the true teacher. It is through the practice of life that I learn everything; and also by practicing yoga nidra and listening to the Lord of Sleep, that I will truly learn how to practice. In this field, only direct experience counts.

PREPARATION (*PRASTUTI*)

Practicing yoga nidra for an hour or more naturally calls for a peaceful place where one will not be disturbed. If possible it should be a silent place, even though noise is not fundamentally a problem in itself. Similarly, if the sensation of cold generates tension, it is better to use a blanket in the beginning, because it is important to be completely still during the session, and preferably in the corpse pose.

DEEP RELAXATION (*SHITHILIKARANA*)

Relaxation is only the means, but not the entire purpose, of the preparatory phase. If one is not relaxed and free of tension, it is impossible to be aware of the profound structures and of the energy, be it during the day or at night. *The more relaxed I am, the more receptive I am.* So here are a few exercises that are easy to select and do at the beginning of a session, in order to let go of physical, emotional, and mental tension.

The "stiffness of the corpse" exercise: just before you take the corpse pose, close your eyes and bring your arms and legs close to the body. Breathe in, hold your breath, and contract the body as much as possible, all the while tightening the arms against the trunk and legs against one another. Observe the body as it stiffens. Then let go of everything as you exhale. Observe the "corpse" as it relaxes and becomes completely still and inert. Who is dying? To whom does this experience appear?

Without intellectualizing, I become aware of my general state, here and now, without trying to change it. For the withdrawal of the senses, I can first listen to the most distant sounds, and gradually bring my attention back to the sounds that are closer to me and inside me, until I come to silence. I become aware of the rise and fall of my breathing by gradually extending my attention to the points pressing down on the floor, from head to toes. With each exhalation, everything settles down, rests, and melts into the silence of the heart center and the sense of touch. I become aware of the vibratory waves, of the mind's space where everything that happens appears and is designed. The eyes remain still, the vision far behind, as a witness, contemplating the infinite depth of this inner sky without comment.

The "wave" exercise: in order to intensify the relaxation and sensitivity, I feel the breath's caress rising in front of my body from my heels to the top of my head when I inhale, and flow downward from the top of my head to my heels and behind the body as I exhale. I observe the rise and fall of my breathing and the waves of sensations that purify me and wash away all my physical and mental tension. Breath after breath, I relish the envelope of sensations and I let go. I allow my body, the shava, to rest and relax to the rhythm of my breathing, which comes and goes like waves on the tranquil ocean.

Here I can visualize the image of Narayana, if it has some significance for me, asleep in his eternal sleep; or Shiva, lying down beneath the goddess Kali. In this way, I allow a new feeling to arise as I inhale; it merges with the vital breath and I allow it to spread throughout the body as I exhale. Anirvan says, "You are not resting in your bed, but on the infinite primordial Ocean of light . . . " With each breath, I become aware of the flow of energy in the spine. Vibration with inhale ("I"), awareness, vibration with exhale ("am"), bliss. The waves of the sensations, emotions, thoughts, and images come and go, but the profound ocean remains perfectly tranquil, a detached spectator to the rise and fall of the waves that appear and disappear in it.

As the practitioner progresses, the relaxation phase will become shorter, especially if a series of postures and breathing exercises has been done beforehand. We can suppose that, in this case, the practitioner is already relaxed, ready, and available.

THE FORCE OF INTENTION (*SANKALPA*)

With this awakened availability and sensitivity, the vibrant energy is felt in one's flesh and bones; our thoughts become creative and give way to intuition. Yoga nidra thus invites us to make a wish or resolve (*sankalpa*), briefly and in a positive way, so as to allow this thought full of energy to appear and take form. I simply inhale, repeat the wish three times with the retention of breath, and I forget it as I exhale. The traditional approach advises us to repeat the same wish until it is fulfilled: all prayers must be repeated at least thrice for the superior forces to hear and fulfill them. It is also possible to inhale with "I . . . " and exhale with the wish in the physical, energetic, and mental structures, one by one, or simultaneously. The wish can also be expressed in the mind's space, between wakefulness and sleep, like a direct message addressed to the subconscious. It can also be formulated in the heart center where the "wish tree" is located, mentioned in texts as the magic tree that fulfills desires: "Resolutions are the wish-granting trees (*kalpataru*); energy (of the mind) is the garden of the trees of plenty."[19]

The wish can also be expressed silently, simultaneously or gradually, at the three levels of the mind's structure: in a way that is articulated, not articulated, or heard. With practice and experience, the wish becomes a nonwish, free of words, thoughts, and intentions. It is a remembering without object, pure presence, without desire or form. There will be no desire other than to remain in the greater Self.

> Abandoning without reserve all desires born of *sankalpa*, and completely restraining the whole group of senses by the mind from all sides.
>
> Little by little, let him attain quietude by his intellect, held firm;

having made the mind established in the Self, let him not think of anything.[20]

Irrespective of the nature of the wish, I remain tranquil, a spectator of everything that appears and disappears.

ROTATION OF CONSCIOUSNESS
(*CHETANA SANCHARANA*)

The rotation of consciousness is an essential phase for reinforcing awareness of oneself and presence to the different structures that compose us, all the while allowing the nonduality of being to awaken through its appeasing power:

An Indian traditional myth says that we have all lost sight of our inner unity. According to this myth, the human being is inhabited by the feeling of having lost something that he knows nothing about, but nevertheless, he would like to find again. This lost taste, closely linked with "conscious vision" is what mythology calls Shiva. As for the desire to find this state of consciousness once again, mythology attributes to it the traits of Shakti, the energy through which Shiva is manifested. These characters represent the two aspects of reality, and when both these aspects are connected, all conflict disappears and there is no more separation. Indian iconography represents them in an indissoluble sexual embrace. It is in the intimacy of this slightly peculiar couple that legend finds its source. The story says that, lost in their union, Shiva and Shakti completely forgot about the universe, in such a way that the balance of the world was in danger. Anxious human beings thus complained about this to the gods, Shiva and Shakti have once again crossed all limits! They decided to carry out a commando operation against them, and some halfhuman halfcelestial beings were appointed to kidnap Shakti at the summit of the Himalayas and hide her on the other side of India, at the Cape Comorin. Once the operation was completed, Shiva slowly came out of his torment and in the blink of an eye (the third one!), he found his companion. Angered that their union had been disturbed, he came to her, grabbed her by the hair and rushed them back to their Himalayan abode. The men, who absolutely did not wish to see them resume their lovemaking, then decided to cut up the goddess into pieces and disperse them in the four corners of the country. As Shiva was dragging his companion, they started cutting up the goddess, first her right thumb, then the second finger, the third, and so on.[21]

In order to fulfill this truly "essential duty" of "collecting the scattered pieces of the goddess" and coming back to the lost unity, I begin by sensing my right thumb.* The rotation can be done on the first three structures, independently or simultaneously, by insisting on the awareness of the sensations of the physical body (skin, muscles, bones and organs), of the vibrations of the energetic body, and the images that naturally appear from the mental body. Thus, after the thumb, I sense each finger, one by one. The flesh, its vibration, and image. Then the palm and back of my hand, my hand and wrist; my forearm up to my elbow and upper arm up to my shoulder; and my whole arm. I then bring my attention to the big right toe, followed by the others; the upper and lower sides of my right foot, my whole foot, heel and ankle; I allow the feeling to move up to my calf, tibia and knee; my thigh, buttock, hip and my whole right leg. I continue in this way with my left leg, then with my left arm. I take the time to feel both my arms and legs together. Then I allow my awareness to come to the base of my body: buttocks, hips, perineum, anus, coccyx, groin, the sacral and sexual region. I am attentive to the sensations and vibrations that appear and disappear. My attention, in this "concentration without tension" continues to climb up

---

*Becoming aware of the right thumb, as compared to other parts of the body, supposedly allows one to rapidly change one's state of consciousness, by its direct action on the brain. See Satyananda, op. cit.

into my stomach, plexus, lumbar region, kidneys, sides; into my chest and back; into the shoulder blades, collarbone, the zones in-between, into the heart and heart center. With each breath, I feel both my legs and torso, up to my shoulders and arms. Then my attention continues to rise up to neck, throat, back of the neck, and cervicals; then into my whole head, brain, and sense organs in the order of the elements.

At last I can taste the found unity by feeling my whole body and its central axis vibrating with each breath in the space of consciousness and in the heart center. I can hear the natural mantra repeating itself through me: "I am," "I am" (*ham'sa*). I am the spectator and the tranquil witness. I make the most of every exhalation to let go and melt into the peaceful background, in my back full of attention, energy, and light. Everything is seen and all phenomena are welcomed, without comments or words. The backdrop observes the coming and going of the worlds, without being affected by it. I am totally aware, lying down like Narayana on an ocean of subtle sensations. The body falls asleep but the consciousness watches over it, like a child falling asleep in his mother's arms.

In order to gather the small bits of energy that are unconscious, the attention can move according to a codified or spontaneous itinerary. The rotation can be external (*bahirnyasa*), centered on the physical body; or it can be internal (*antaranyasa*), centered on the wheels of energy or the appearance of images. As mentioned above, this movement can also be done simultaneously in the first three "sheaths" by becoming aware of the sensation, vibration, and image. It can be done according to different orders and directions. It is important to feel what is happening without allowing the mind to wander off into associations. For this to happen, apart from knowing the itinerary and not having to think about it, you can use the heartbeat, the breath, or a short mantra such as *AUM* or *RAM* to "touch" a particular body part in order to localize it, feel it, and let it go. Each "touch" is like making an offering. In this way, knowing what is held on to makes it easier to let it go. This is why once the body is deeply felt, it can fade away. It disappears into the void along with the sense of "me." Only the peaceful and silent taste of conscious sleep remains. This rotation of consciousness can also designate a pilgrimage to "the places where the pieces of the goddess fell and where temples have been erected."*[22] I myself have tasted this lost unity by traveling in India from one holy place to another, just like I do in my body, from one limb to another. An old proverb from the *Skanda Purana* guided me on the path to four holy places, to try to collect what I thought was lost knowledge: "To see Chidambaram, to be born in Thiruvarur, to die in Varanasi or to remember Arunachala, all of these alone will confer Liberation." If this old verse guided my way, yoga nidra allowed me to be present to the links between the places, and to the fact that in the absolute there is only one link and one sacred space in which all separations are absorbed. The energy centers, represented as points in the body or sacred places, unite in the awareness. Everything appears in me and I remain still. First, I see everything that is not a link, and then I die, fade away, and allow the link to be born to the awareness, to remember it and live in it, by being the spectator who is free from everything that passes by.

THE COUNTDOWN

In order to observe the mind's process and the space in which this occurs, it is possible to let oneself go with a countdown, starting from the 108th, 54th, or 27th breath. Inhale and exhale 108, inhale and exhale 107, and so on, down to zero, which is at the center of each one of us. With each exhalation, the counting dissolves into silence and I am a spectator to the countdown. I allow it to happen and come undone, all by itself and without interfering. I allow myself to be car-

---

*Many ancient texts, like the Puranas (which include *Shiva, Devi, Brahmanda, Kalika, Mahapitha*), the *Pithanirnaya Tantra* or the *Shakti Pitha Strotram* of Shankaracharya mention 18, 52, 64, or 108 "places of force" (*shakti pitha*), which refer to different body parts. The places and the story line may vary according to the sources, but the profound meaning is always the same.

ried into the unknown. I just am happy counting backward, going from the multiple toward the one. This is the perfect moment in which to fall asleep, without falling into total oblivion. But it is also a phase in which I might fall asleep completely, and fall into total oblivion. So, I must be alert . . .

The countdown can also be an opportunity to purify the space of the mind by alternative breathing, without blocking my nostrils with my fingers: I inhale through the left nostril and exhale through the right nostril, inhale with right nostril, exhale with the left one, and so on. I simply become aware of my breath moving on one side, then on the other, in a manner that can feel very tactile.

Arriving at zero creates a pause in the fluctuations of the mind and allows for an opening, perfect for feeling wonder and joy and conducive to exploration.

WORKING WITH THEMES

The initial phases of the session are meant to create total availability for more intense practice between wakefulness and sleep. By juggling with the different bodies, sheaths, centers, structures, and other phenomena, it is possible to compose a very large number of practices for exploring the inner labyrinth, and perhaps discovering a way out of suffering and ignorance. The core of the practice involves all the limbs of yoga, especially concentration, meditation, and profound contemplation. Irrespective of the theme that is chosen (such as death, the five elements, and so on) and the original intention, it must all end by dissolving in the deep peace of silence.

Most yoga nidra sessions are essentially based on fundamentally existential questions. Some aim to observe the different structures in detail and from different angles, with their processes, links, and transitions: the physical body and its tissues (skin, muscles, bones, organs), the sensory system and its relationship with the unconscious, the energetic body (centers, supports, breathing, meridians, and so on), and the different aspects of thought (mind, memory, intelligence, and sense of "me"), the way in which they appear and disappear, and so on. If yoga nidra systematically invites us to attentively observe sensations, vibrations, light, and sound, some practices can concentrate on one of these in particular by introducing breathing exercises and mantras. Among the important themes, yoga nidra does not forget to question our relationship with animality, time, the future, desires, the elements, pleasure, ecstasy, love, the sense of "me," the divine, dream, sleep, and death.

Generally speaking, the sequence always evolves according to the ascending order of the energy centers, like we do in the practice of postures. Once the countdown is over, it gives a direction to the session. Furthermore, according to traditional teachings, this order coincides with the diminution of the senses and the dissolution of the elements in the processes of sleep and death. This general search divides the process and constitutes excellent preparation. Here is a broad outline, which can be adapted in a variety of ways:

I start by becoming aware of the energy center at the base, at the level of my coccyx, uniting breathing and thought (*ham'sa*, "I am" . . .) with the sensation of vibration. This will allow me to strengthen my concentration and sensitivity, as well as open up to a new space. I might even perceive physical and energetic particularities (like tissues, wheels, forms, colors, and so on), in a more or less detailed manner. What is of utmost importance is the feeling or the sensation. I use every breath to allow the close link between the energy center and the other structures to appear, and I feel the connection: the anus, the sense of smell, and the impressions left by it; the tissues of the physical body and its inertia, its stability, its solid state, its relation with the earth element, and with the feeling of tranquility. Like Narayana or Shiva, I am only a witness to the phenomena that appear and disappear, and to the changing states, without comment or appraisal, and without getting carried away by the energy of their movements. The breath stretches out. I am open to the scent of presence.

I then allow myself to slip into the pelvic region, at the level of the sacral region. With each breath, I become aware of the connection between the sexual organs, the sense of taste, the water element, the blood and energy circulation, the waves of vibration in my whole body, beyond the skin. I allow a feeling of fluidity and joy to arise. A new taste.

My attention continues to climb into the stomach, in level with the lumbar spine. I explore the connections between the solar plexus, the fire element, the sense of sight, shapes, my eyes, the heat, light, vibrations, emotions, the mind, and dreams. With each breath, I sink deeply into a vibratory emanation. From Narayana's belly emerges a lotus flower on which Lord Brahma is seated, creating thoughts and worlds that rise and fall. Beauty is the taste of reality. Breath after breath, the fire consumes desires, fears, and the sense of "me." The interval between wakefulness and sleep is approaching.

My attention then climbs into the heart center, at the level of the dorsal spine: skin, hands, the air element, the sense of touch, sleep, and "me," on the brink of the Void. With every breath, the "I" disappears into a feeling of expansion, a sensation of impersonal energy, free as air, which spreads and envelopes the whole universe, beyond the limits of the skin and the mind. It is the taste of beatitude and love. "The child sleeps but the Mother is watching over him."

My attention then goes to the throat center and the cervicals: ears, vocal cords, the sense of hearing, the space element, and the sound, which is the last link between the *dying* and the phenomenal world. The feeling of expansion gives way to total stillness. The expansion itself, like breath, appears in the void. It is the taste of silence.

Then my attention moves to the forehead center, between the eyebrows, in the middle of my head. The physical space appears in this mental space made up of conscious energy, like all the centers and elements. It is the taste of awareness and pure joy.

Finally, this mental space itself appears in the space of awareness. The energy ends its race in the center of a thousand petals, in the union of the void above the head with the void in the heart. It is the union of clarity and vacuity. It is the taste of Being, of the Uncreated, and of found unity.

> I Am *Brahman*, of the nature of pure Consciousness, without qualities, free from Ignorance, free from the three states of waking, dream and deep sleep. Living in all beings like the ether, I am the witness free from all their defects.[23]

Sensations, emotions, and thoughts, as well as the states of wakefulness, dream, and sleep, appear and disappear like clouds in the sky, but the sky of consciousness remains perfectly still, unaffected and unchanging. It contains everything and permeates everything; it is everything. Ramana Maharshi used to say, "The whole universe is in the body and the whole body is in the Heart. So the universe is contained in the Heart. . . . Heart is Thy Name, O Lord!" Like Swami Dayananda so rightly puts it, "There is not only one God, there is only God." At this stage, no more practice is possible. It is no longer a question of effort, concentration, action, or intention. There is nobody left; only Awareness remains.

VISUALIZATIONS

A typical yoga nidra session also includes particular visualizations that can be practiced independently. Some schools systematically use images in their sequences and even transform them into stories and scenarios. If such practices can allow us to access the deeper levels of individual and collective subconscious, like intuition for example, they can also overstimulate ordinary associative thoughts instead of pausing them, thus preventing us from awakening to the reality beyond this mechanical structure. It is up to each individual to practice with care, sincerity, and attention, and see what works the best. Such practices can also be a good support for dream yoga.

The images that are used in these types of sessions are often symbols and archetypes; they can be yoga postures, divine representations, trees, flowers, animals, birds, mountains, oceans, and anything related to nature such as day, night, and the seasons. They can be logically selected according to the five elements (earth, water, fire, air, and space), or according to other themes like love, emptiness, sleep, and death.

The classical texts of yoga, Vedanta, and Tantra are full of these images for the awakening of a finer quality of feeling and intuition, and thus an inspiration for yoga nidra. For example, the *Shiva Samhita* mentions images that symbolically represent the human body composed of the five elements: "In this body, the mount Meru—i.e., the vertebral column—is surrounded by seven islands; there are rivers, seas, mountains, fields; and lords of the fields too. There are in it seers and sages; all the stars and planets as well. There are sacred pilgrimages, shrines; and presiding deities of the shrines. The sun and moon, agents of creation and destruction, also move in it. Ether, air, water and earth are also there."[24] Thus, by allowing these images to spontaneously appear in or around me, in the wordless space without commentary, without associating knowledge or any thought to it, I can feel them resonate intuitively in specific parts of the body like the spine, the energy centers, and the principal meridians. What is important is to perceive and know things in a different way, without the usual filter of discursive thoughts, and to remain in this subtle feeling. Therefore, in a session with many images, it is important to allow them to pass by quickly (or to mention them quickly, if you are conducting the session), so that the mind does not take over and start commenting on them. With a little practice, I can visualize a complete series of images as I exhale, slowly and deeply, or in rhythm with my sleeper's breathing, repeating this as many times as required. This exercise can also be practiced several times during the day (or at night), irrespective of whether I am sitting, standing, lying down, or walking, or with open or closed eyes. In the end, what is important is that the image should bring me back to the space of tranquility and awareness in which it appears. It is not about speculating on phenomena or knowing; it's about diving into the heart, and simply being.

MERGING WITH THE HEART

When a particular yoga practice succeeds in stopping the fluctuations of the mind, it instantly becomes useless and impossible to do; useless because there is nothing to do, and impossible because there is no one to do it. The ego or the sense of "me" is erased, along with the thoughts. All that remains is the taste of silence and the void, the indescribable joy of the original vision, which is impersonal and intensely alive. In the case of a formal session, this moment of pure meditation will be presented as a long moment of silence. It directly opens up to intuition, beatitude, and the blissful witness of this epiphany, to the bliss of the self and the permanent awareness of the "I":

> In the centre of the Heart-cave there shines alone the one Brahman as the "I-I," the Atman. Reach the Heart by diving deep in quest of the Self, or by controlling the mind with the breath, and stay established in the Atman.[25]

> The void is the Consciousness reflecting itself, perceiving that it is distinct and saying "I am not that (*neti neti*)." This is the highest state attained by yogis.[26]

RESOLVE (*SANKALPA*) AND FINAL PHASE (*SAMAPTI*)

In the case of a formal session, this moment is perfect to hear one's resolve or wish three times—the same one that was made at the beginning of the session. From this bliss without form will emerge the verb, the wish, sound, light, and vibration, and they will then appear in the guise of the world. As soon as the wish fades away in the vibrant void, I gradually become aware of the different structures leading to the physical body, one by one, from head to toe. I thus remain a motionless spectator of the body that is moving once again.* I take my

---

*What does not change and what remains still when the body and mind begin to move again and their state changes?

time to enjoy this by remaining in the luminous presence to myself, which, through practice and grace, extends little by little to the other moments of my days and nights, with the profound feeling of being happy, tranquil, and free. I am. This manner of coming out of a session is also applicable to the moment when you wake up in the morning and to the appearance of the sense of "me." A complete practice can consist in preparing and observing the process of falling sleep with the different phases of a regular practice session, until one falls asleep in the heart. In this way, each time you wake up, it becomes an opportunity to simply observe the transition or to continue the practice that you were doing. Or you can simply remain a spectator to the passing states . . . until you wake up and remember your resolve or wish; then, after a moment of awareness, your body will start to move, get out of bed, and do its daily activities.

The Art of Living in Total Awareness

Yoga nidra is not limited to formal practices and the observation of sleep. It is an integral approach to all states of consciousness. It offers a methodology that varies from one school to another, but more than anything, yoga nidra is an outlook, a way of being, and an art of living every day, which has nothing to do with appearances, morals, or the nature of activities. It is not a substitute for any other practice, but can be practiced in addition to all activities, in the union of total awareness and deep peace. This sacred link can be established by recognizing the silence of sleep during wakefulness. "We have only to invoke this wakeful silence and expand our consciousness into it, spreading it into the Yoga-heart of the Mother. In this way even sleep can be transformed."[27]

As soon as I begin to wake up, I can use the interval between sleep and waking to go straight into meditation, whether formal or casual. I am open, without any intention, and I allow this silence to welcome phenomena, my first actions and events of the day, and my social, professional, and family obligations. It is not about changing one's life conditions, but about observing oneself reacting to these very conditions. True meditation is not an action in the sense that meditation is not something that can be *done,* it is simply *being,* and can therefore easily be practiced in addition to my daily activities. That being said, it is important to make the time to sit in silence at least twice a day, because this silence needs to be recognized and cultivated.

I prepare to experience my daily activities with awareness by making the time to sit and meditate for a predetermined period. All the limbs of yoga participate in this exercise. Seated in a comfortable position, with one hand on top of the other, I start by relaxing my whole body, from the head to the toes, one body part after the other. With each breath I allow the tension to come undone. I then bring my attention to my natural breathing, without trying to change it. I am happy observing the air coming in and going out, with brief pauses in between. Breath after breath, I allow my senses to withdraw by becoming aware of the sound of my breath (*ham'sa*), of the silence in the pauses between breaths, and of the silent background in which breathing takes place. I concentrate on my breathing, allowing the mind's agitation to come and die in the silence. Once the tranquility of my body and mind are established, I start observing the sensations from head to toes, starting at the fontanel and moving the attention from one part to another, and then back from my toes to my head. I make sure that I am alert and equanimous in the face of every sensation, emotion, or thought that appears, so as to not react with desire or aversion. Who am I? Who is observing? Slowly but surely, the perception of phenomena strengthens the tranquil and silent space in which it appears. By remaining in pure observation, thoughts are finally paused and consciousness withdraws itself and awakens to its true nature: "I am." Meditation thus becomes contemplation without object, without knowing, without knowledge and remembering, without technique or intention. There is no longer anybody who thinks he knows, who thinks he is doing something or meditating. All that remains is consciousness and the joy of being, a feeling of impersonal peace and unlimited love. When the meditation ends, I can take a few minutes to let the peace and subtle vibrations spread to the whole universe, like a wish I am sharing with sincerity and benevolence: "May all beings be peaceful and happy." *AUM*. Later, if I am caught up in the flow of phenomena when I get back to my activities, the slightest awareness of any agitation, tension, or negativity should make me come back to this silent observation, *here and now:*

> If only you will remain resting in consciousness, seeing yourself as distinct from the body, then even now you will become happy, peaceful and free from bonds.[28]

ELECTRICITY DOES NOT DIE WHEN THE BULB IS BROKEN

A direct and instantaneous method to achieve Jivanmukti, bypassing the aforesaid methods has been propounded by Ashtavakra thus:

Have first that firm conviction that I am NOT the Body-mind complex. Know well that you are as separate from the body as electricity is from the bulb. Hence, the limitations of the body (death, old age, disease, sufferings etc.) do not apply to your Self. The electrical energy inside a bulb can never be destroyed. So, let one practice sitting for a few hours each day absolutely relaxed and not necessarily in any particular posture, in the garden or some place of solitude free from all distractions of visitors (including mobile or other telephones etc. used in modern times). Be aware of nothing else except the feeling of bare existence and being alive i.e., "I am." Be happy in that feeling. Do not think of the body and do not add any qualification to the feeling of 'amness', such as, "I am a woman," "I am aged 30 years," "I am an Indian," "I am an Engineer," "I am having headache" etc. Simply "BE." If your eyes are open, do not see things specifically or distinguish the objects. Do not distinguish various noises. Remain in the totality of an uncritical, unjudging, undistinguishing and undifferentiated perception.

Do not think "I am." Just remain in the consciousness i.e., the feeling of your existence, like a new born child which has no vocabulary to think but revels in its pulsating existence. If one can permanently remain in this state (which can be attained through practice), here and now one can get Jivanmukti.[29]

Fields of Application for Yoga Nidra

Consciousness of being and Delight of being are the first parents. Also, they are the last transcendences.

SRI AUROBINDO

Unlike modern popular methods, the aim of yoga nidra is not at all materialistic. It is neither a technique of personal development and well-being, nor is it a hobby or coaching, generally based on strengthening a certain self-confidence related to the sense of ego. Even practicing for good health is not a goal in itself, although it is clearly a positive side effect of the practice. The aim of yoga nidra is above all a spiritual one, related to knowing the Self, liberation from suffering, and realization of one's true nature. That being said, to recognize the different structures of the being implies completely letting go, which has a positive influence on the psycho-physiological dimension—the body and mind—thus benefiting our health in general. In this way, knowing oneself is by nature deeply therapeutic. And by strengthening the faculty of discrimination (*viveka*), benevolence, and openness, it is also profoundly social, humane, and creative.

By teaching me to live in the present moment, yoga nidra allows me to see the dimensions of time and of the mind in a new way. Observing this reveals the energies that operate behind the phenomena that compose my destiny, and then perhaps I can have a better understanding of the events that happen to me and the situations that repeat themselves day after day. This attentive observation allows me to reconcile my past, no matter what it was, and welcome the future, no matter what happens. For if stress, anxiety, and fear are often the causes of numerous diseases, the fear of death is very much at the source of all fears. And by dispelling this fear at the source of all others, yoga nidra also participates in preserving general health and well-being.

By preserving one from stress, anxiety, depression, and fear, deep relaxation slows down the deterioration of the immune system and the development of psychosomatic pathologies. And by inundating the body with a feeling of happiness that emerges from the awareness of being, the practice strengthens our health at the very heart of our cells. This positive action and blueprint of the physical body as an experienced reality have thus become the two most important principles of sophrology. This method developed by neuropsychiatrist Alfonso Caycedo in the 1960s is considerably inspired by Indian philosophies and by phenomenology. In addition to the influence of Sri Aurobindo's integral yoga, practical Sophrology is highly inspired by yoga nidra, not only with regard to the sequence of the techniques, but also the way in which the session is conducted orally and the search for that state of consciousness between waking and sleeping. With its numerous social and preventive fields of applications, I believe that this modern method of sophrology based on body awareness and a phenomenological attitude is a therapeutic extension of yoga nidra. Relaxing, letting go, and becoming aware can generate energies that are important for the health of the body and the mind, for the feeling of well-being and vitality, for concentration, creativity, and the quality of sleep.

A session focused on the therapeutic aspect follows the same sequence as a regular one, but with a different intention. Here is an example. With synchronized breath, the preparatory phase will pay particular attention to relaxation, letting go of the tensions in the body and in the mind, with awareness of the whole body, its heat, and its vital energy. The resolve or wish occupies an important place here, in the sense that it sends a positive and embodied suggestion to the subconscious, a wish that can easily be adapted to different pathologies. If one has the time—and according to one's experience—the rotation of consciousness on the physical body, which is generally just a quick verification or a scan, can go into more detail: into the skin, muscles, bones, and different vital organs. I allow the attention, the life, to touch every single point and invigorate it, with full awareness of my breathing. I take the time to feel the plexus, brain, and spinal cord when I inhale, and I allow the pure happiness to saturate my cells as I exhale. I become aware of the vitality, vigor, joy of being, centers, and waves of energy circulating in my body. The breath and the inner rhythm balance each other out and I become aware of my heart and the energy that makes it beat. With this feeling I can try to relieve some pain in the body by drowning it in the space of a vaster sensation, for example, or by expelling it when I exhale. I can also stimulate or appease a tissue by drawing on a warm or cool energy in one of the energy centers (or elsewhere) as I inhale, and then allow it to diffuse to specific body parts as I exhale. By attentively renewing this experience several times, a feeling of relief can be established. The countdown exercise can be used to sink into peace and sensitivity, freeing intuition; and maybe you can allow a situation to appear toward the end of the countdown, a kind of sensory vision, in which the problems have been either solved or accepted with joy and serenity. Then, beyond all images and the mind, in the "heart-cave," that unaffected peace always remains, a profound silence in which the cells regenerate and the body rests. To conclude a session, it is enough to mentally repeat your resolve or wish three times and then allow the force of yoga and the energy of attention to incarnate it as you become aware of your body once again. Take a moment to revel in the taste and feel bathed in joy and gratitude.

In absolute terms, yoga nidra does not try to change the course of things, but helps us to see and accept reality as it is, by uniting with it at every moment. "If something happens, it's good. If it does not happen, it's also good." This acceptance does not prevent me from trying to do anything, but such efforts should be made without being attached to the action and its results. In the same way, true acceptance can never come from dualistic thought. Thoughts will resign, but will never give up; there will always be a *yes, but* followed by suffering. When in fact, acceptance is *yes* without *but;* acceptance is welcoming the situation quietly without desiring it to be anything other than what it is. By observing the part of myself that does not accept, by giving it space, it is possible for me to awaken to the benevolent space of acceptance, beyond thoughts; I can recognize that if "I-me" does not accept things the way they are, the vast silence that I am welcomes everything without distinction, but moreover with love. Then everything becomes simpler. Here and now, the very observation reveals itself to be the supreme cure. In the case of pain—a headache for instance—I say, "My head is hurting," talking about myself. But the witness is different from the one who is seen in suffering. The witness is not the one who is suffering.[30] If I realize this when I am sick, I am happy and instantly cured of everything.

The Ultimate Surrender

"It is necessary to be awake all day long, in order to sleep well" Nietzsche wrote in *Thus Spake Zarathustra*. In the context of yoga nidra, this affirmation takes on a new meaning and is like a teaching of great importance. And we can also add that it is up to us to sleep well at night, in order to be truly awake.

Yoga nidra thus offers a path of relaxation, inner knowledge, discharge, regeneration, and opening up to spaces free of suffering, be it in wakefulness, in life, in sleep, or in death. By invading the unawareness at the source of all conditioning, yoga nidra allows for a new outlook on the world, on others, and on oneself—an outlook that is more peaceful. With regular training on a daily basis, the practices fall into place on their own, even at night. Everything is clear and luminous: a new flavor that changes life, our way of knowing ourselves, and of being.

The philosophy is essentially practical. The knowing and the being are reunited in a harmonious, benevolent, and nourishing dance. The map is not the territory, but it allows us to move forward on the path, to lose ourselves then to find ourselves; it lets us be seized by what "is neither lost nor found."

I can relax without practicing yoga nidra, but I cannot practice yoga nidra without being relaxed just like in meditation. In wakefulness, the relaxation essentially operates on the level of the physical body and its tissues. If I am not relaxed and am completely tensed it is impossible to be aware, whether at day or at night, of the profound structures and of the energy that circulates in them. Whereas in the practice of conscious sleep, the deeper the relaxation, the more available and open I become. Even though it is only a preparatory phase it is still very important because perceiving tensions allows me to let go of them and awaken to a space of consciousness that is ever peaceful and tensionless. The different processes are observed peacefully. The transition and intervals are observed and the inquiry continues: "Who am I? Sensations appear and disappear inside me, so I am not this tensed or relaxed body, healthy or sick. Emotions appear and disappear in me, so I am thus not these changing emotions. Thoughts appear and disappear in me, so I am thus not these thoughts. To whom do these thoughts appear?" The only possible answer would be "I am," but if an answer appears to me, it means that in reality I am prior to it. In the light of this witnessing presence, the ego, the "I-thought," suddenly appears to be a simple tension of the mind, the crystallization of a thought that belongs to no one, a knot that lacks firmness, and a contraction that no longer exists once it is released, like in the heart of deep sleep, meditation, or conscious sleep. But it is necessary to remain alert because the states are changing and the tensions may come back without my noticing them.

With practice, yoga nidra, as a reality and not as a means, reveals itself to be the ever peaceful background of all my activities and all my experiences. Conscious or unconscious, being or not being, tensed or relaxed, asleep or awake: all these dualities end up dissolving into that which is neither this nor that. No form of yoga as a technique or a practice can allow me to realize the Self, because realizing the Self is not an action. Yoga nidra, on the other hand, can make me available to such a discovery by familiarizing me with the non-Self and awakening me to a different quality of listening. Through the total commitment and conscious effort that are required against the mechanical manifestations of my person, it produces the friction through which noneffort sets in, like a transparent and clear truth, vibrant and luminous all at once. When all concepts are dissolved, the yogi disappears in the transparent benevolence of his true nature that is the same Consciousness in all of us, the unique underlying Force in each one of our multiple eccentricities and the Life at work in each one of our cells. Like in all traditional paths, yoga nidra invites us to realize, by simple observation, that we are not the bulb, but the electricity, and that the electricity is the same in each bulb. Moreover, that electricity does not die when the bulb burns out.

But, as soon as there is light, the bulb easily tends to think that the current comes from it and that it is producing the light. I must be very alert not to get caught up in the illusion of the "me" that latches on and gives itself credit for everything, if it reappears. Ramana Maharshi urges us to differentiate "the temporary stillness of thought," which is a result of concentration and temporarily arresting the movement of thoughts. "As soon as this concentration ceases, thoughts, old and new, rush in as usual; and even if this temporary lulling of mind should last a thousand years, it will never lead to total destruction of thought, which is what is called liberation from birth and death. The practitioner must therefore be ever on the alert and enquire within as to who has this experience, who realizes its pleasantness."[31] If I can experience the peace, the silence, and the void, it means that I am still beyond this sensation or feeling. One must not be deluded by a false sense of liberation and be fooled by such periods of silence and thought. On the contrary, it is at this moment that one must become alert again and look inside with a lot of attention to realize who experiences this silence. For there is no beginning and no end to the silence of the Self, which never changes.

Only thoughts appear and disappear. Ramana Maharshi says, "The true 'I' is not apparent and the false 'I' is parading itself. This false 'I' is the obstacle to your right knowledge. Find out from where this false 'I' arises. Then it will disappear. You will then be only what you are, that is, absolute being." Therefore, it is not enough to simply stop thoughts in order to be free; it is absolutely necessary to recognize their source.

Yoga nidra is not a technique to be practiced, a method to learn, a faculty to develop, an intention, an experience, a state, or a goal to accomplish. Yoga nidra is simply recognizing what I have always been, even before knowing that "I am." I can thus sing and celebrate the Glory of Being with Shankaracharya:

> There is no waking state for me nor dream or deep sleep.
>
> I am not the Self identified with the experience of the waking state, nor identified with dream state, nor identified with deep sleep.
>
> I am really the Fourth (Turiya). That One, the Residue, the Auspicious, the Alone, I am Shiva.
>
> I do not have fear of death, as I do not have death.
>
> I have no separation from my true self, no doubt about my existence, nor have I discrimination on the basis of birth.
>
> I have no father or mother, nor did I have a birth.
>
> I am not the relative, nor the friend, nor the guru, nor the disciple.
>
> I am That eternal knowing and bliss, love and pure consciousness, I am Shiva, I am Shiva.[32]

PART III

PUTTING YOGA NIDRA INTO PRACTICE

Four Practice Sessions and 115 Micro-Practices

In order to be able to practice yoga nidra without the presence of a teacher, you can record your own voice and then use it to experience these sessions in a guided manner. The ellipses or suspension points indicate short or long moments of silence, according to one's intention. The art of conducting these sessions lies in measuring these pauses in a way that will bring growing awareness. With practice, the moments of silence—which are not moments of absence, but of presence—become longer. You can note that the use of the wish or resolve (*sankalpa*) is neither necessary nor systematic. You can adapt the position for practicing in order to be more comfortable by using a cushion, a blanket, and a scarf to cover your eyes.

SESSION 1

Blue Star
(Nilatara Yoga Nidra)

During a visit to Rishikesh, I was very lucky to meet remarkable yogis belonging to the lineage of the visionary sages of ancient India and the Himalayan masters, of which Swami Rama and Swami Veda Bharati are eminent representatives. Having met a direct disciple of the latter, I was able to discover and study a form of yoga nidra that I had never experienced before. This once again reminded me of the importance of oral transmission in yoga nidra, in India and in Tibet, and how it is impossible to limit this ancestral practice, whose source is lost in the dawn of time, to a particular founder, school of thought, or form of practice. Like the Upanishads, yoga nidra is literally and essentially studied when one *sits down* or *lies down* at the Master's feet. The teaching I received in Rishikesh, inspired by Vedic tradition and centered on the art of dying, is very similar to the tantric teachings of Shaivism that I had received from the traditional *natha yogis* of Varanasi (Banaras), except for a few minor details. This Himalayan approach aims to have full awareness of the sensations, emotions, thoughts, dreams, and deep sleep in order to recognize the ever peaceful witness of these different states and experiences. By conducting scientific experiments, Swami Rama proved, for example, that yoga nidra allows one to consciously stabilize in the delta waves that the brain emits during deep sleep. Swami Rama could also control the involuntary muscles of his physical body such as his heart, which he could slow down until it stopped completely. But this type of performance and laboratory experiments have little importance and are conducted only to satisfy the curiosity of the agitated and anxious mind and its constant need for proof. In fact, yoga nidra gives importance to the physical body only at the beginning of the session, during the relaxation phase, or in a therapeutic approach. The practice rapidly helps one experience full awareness of the subtle energetic network that inhabits and surrounds the gross body. There can be no yoga nidra without a deep understanding of the energetic system and the mind's processes, and the feeling and knowing that they are the stepping-stones to higher awareness. Thus, every step of the way the practitioner, knowing what he is holding on to, can let go of it; he can set aside the objects and the alleged subject of the experience and allow them both to dissolve in the luminous void of Consciousness, just like Narayana lying down in eternal yoga nidra:

Yoga Nidra is experiencing the state of consciousness that God has when there is no universe. God does not depend on the universe, the universe depends on God. The mind does not depend on the body, the body depends on the mind. For now, Yoga Nidra should be practiced in *shavasana*. Swami Rama says that *shavasana* is one of the most advanced postures. People think it's just lying down. God's position is one of the most advanced postures, because in the God's posture you make a transition from physical postures to mental exercises. God's posture is the link from *jagrat,* from wakeful state, to mastering dream, sleep and Yoga Nidra. The two levels of Yoga Nidra, the measurable one where the laboratory machines are showing that your brain is producing delta brain waves; it is the slowest brain wave, around 1 to 4 hertz per second; that part can be measured. But what the mind is experiencing, that cannot be measured. So I go back to the same grounds again, first understanding the consciousness at the transcendental and cosmological level, as a philosophy. In all the Sanskrit texts on Yoga Nidra, Yoga Nidra is said to be that state of divine consciousness. Then, learning the methods and exercises that are preparatory to Yoga Nidra. So now, the third state, experiencing Yoga Nidra, the measurable part and the immeasurable part. Using that immeasurable part of your personal experience to verify the philosophy that you have been taught, that yes, the philosophy is correct. Because all spiritual philosophies have come from somebody's personal experience of higher states of consciousness. When you believe in somebody's statement about that consciousness, you follow a religion. But here, we are not following a religion. When you test that philosophy by practical methods of spirituality, that is called yoga. So out of that experience, you check and verify that what the ancient rishis and the texts and the masters have said, yes, yes, it is correct. Now remember one point: you may use the same pathways for going into meditation, and you may use the same pathways for going into Yoga Nidra. This is a very important point. You may use the same pathways for going into meditation, and you may use the same pathways for going into Yoga Nidra. In the tradition of the Himalayan masters that we follow, when you are going into meditation, you are using your *mantra* with your breath. When you are going into Yoga Nidra, you are not using any other thought, but only the feel of the flow, not even the *mantra*. That is one of the major differences between the pathways of meditation and the pathways of Yoga Nidra. Now, I am not going to give you a long lecture on the chakra system. We are talking of states of consciousness. Now, the center of *jagrat,* wakeful state, is in the eyebrow center. The center for the control of the dream state is in the throat center. The control of the sleep state is in the heart center. The control of the immune systems and the *prana* field is in the navel center. And so on. So, as I said, these *kriyas* help you at many different levels. For example, as I said, the throat center can help you control your eating and drinking. Lots of people are reading books about guided dreams. If you go to sleep with the image of the stainless full moon in the throat center, you will learn to master the dream state. Now it makes a difference whether you are concentrating on a white moon, or you are concentrating on a slightly pale moon. I cannot initiate you into all of this in just one night. What you have learnt in these sessions, practice, practice, practice . . .[1]

According to the rishi yoga school of thought, yoga nidra is also considered to be an excellent therapeutic tool for problems related to sleep, stress, blood pressure, memory, or restlessness of the mind and emotions. But for the yogi, yoga nidra is practiced primarily to know the Self, for Samadhi, and for going beyond the states of wakefulness, dream, and sleep, as well as beyond life and death. Like the natha yoga tradition, the rishi yoga tradition also considers death as the main theme for the serious practitioner. Both schools insist on relaxation, full awareness of the body, of the energy fields, and states of consciousness, the importance of the expansion of the heart center and of silence, and how to maintain this quality of attention in every moment of daily life.

For example, here is a basic practice, the "corpse journey" (*shava yatra*) or the "blue star" (*nila tara*) practice, which aims to purify the energy centers through sixty-one specific points where three nadis (*marma*) or more than three nadis (chakras) meet. Due to stress and negativity, tensions, knots, or blockages appear in these places. This fundamental session allows one to surpass the physical level (*shthula sharira*) and navigate in the energetic and subtle structure (*sukshma sharira*), allowing the knots to come undone and the vital energy (prana) to circulate freely and in a correct way. This subtle realization induces a very deep state of relaxation and openness, conducive to the recognition of the Presence and joy that are inherent to it. But like an Indian proverb says, "to know the taste of milk, you must drink milk."

The practice will be all the more effective if it is done after a hatha yoga session or after a meditative walk. This helps the cells to regenerate and gets rid of the most visible tensions. The body will thus be energized, alert, and ready for deep relaxation.

∽

The Practice

PREPARATION

Lie down on your stomach in crocodile pose (*makarasana*) with your forehead resting on your forearms (left hand on the right elbow and right hand on the left elbow), legs slightly apart with your feet pointing outward . . . close your eyes . . . and become aware of the gravity of your body . . . and of your abdominal breathing . . . the abdomen rises as you breathe in . . . falls as your breathe out . . . allow the body to relax . . . let your breath flow freely, without pauses . . . [Practice this exercise for about five minutes or the time needed for the abdominal breathing to set in].

Be totally aware of your breath and of your body, be attentive to any change in your position and of the transition from one pose to another . . . Then, turn over to lie down on your back, in corpse pose (*shavasana*), arms and legs slightly apart from the body, palms facing upward, feet turned outward, back straight . . . Promise yourself that you will not move during the entire session . . .

RELAXATION

Become aware of the floor on which you are lying down . . . of the space that your body occupies on the floor, from head to toe . . . of the subtle movement of your stomach rising and falling to the rhythm of your breathing . . . mentally, draw a mandala of three circles of light around yourself . . . and decide that your mind will neither leave this mandala, nor allow anything to enter it . . . observe your body surrounded by the circle of light . . . your breath, your stomach rising and falling . . . relax your mind . . . bring your attention to the top of your head and relax your whole head and forehead . . . your eyebrows, your eyelids, your eyes, and eyeballs . . . relax your nostrils . . . your cheeks . . . your lips, mouth, and tongue . . . your chin . . . your neck, back of the neck, and your throat . . . relax your right shoulder . . . the shoulder joint . . . the upper arm and the elbow . . . forearm, your wrist . . . the back of your hand, your palm . . . your right thumb . . . right index finger, middle finger, ring finger, and little finger . . . the tips of your fingers . . . every joint . . . your palm, the back of your hand . . . your wrist . . . forearm, elbow . . . upper arm up to the shoulder joint . . . relax your shoulder completely . . . your neck and neck joints . . . the base of your throat . . . relax your left shoulder and shoulder joint . . . your upper arm up to the elbow . . . your forearm, wrist . . . the back of your hand, your palm . . . your thumb . . . index finger, middle finger, ring finger, and little finger . . . your fingertips . . . your palm, the back of your hand . . . your wrist . . . your forearm, your elbow . . . your upper arm up to the shoulder joint . . .

your neck and neck joint . . . the base of your throat . . . your chest . . . your ribs, under your armpits, and under your ribs . . . your chest . . . your back . . . the heart region . . . your stomach . . . around your stomach . . . your navel . . . lower abdomen . . . waist . . . hips . . . relax your right thigh and all its muscles . . . your knee . . . your calf . . . your right ankle . . . right foot . . . each toe, starting with the big toe . . . the sole of your foot, your heel . . . right ankle, calf . . . your whole knee . . . your thigh . . . your right hip joint . . . your pelvis . . . your left hip joint . . . left thigh . . . your whole left knee . . . calf . . . left ankle . . . left foot . . . each toe, starting with the big toe . . . the sole of your left foot, your left heel . . . left ankle . . . calf . . . your whole knee . . . your thigh . . . the left hip joint . . . pelvis . . . your hips . . . waist . . . lower abdomen . . . navel . . . stomach . . . feel your whole stomach . . . relax all your inner organs . . . the heart center . . . rib cage, chest . . . your lungs and chest . . . your armpits . . . back . . . shoulders and shoulder joints . . . your upper arms, elbows, forearms . . . your wrists, hands . . . your thumbs, index fingers, middle fingers, ring fingers, and little fingers . . . your fingertips . . . your palms . . . wrists . . . forearms, elbows . . . upper arms, shoulder joints, and shoulders . . . your whole neck, the base of your throat, the Adam's apple, inside your throat, and the base of your tongue . . . relax your tongue, your chin, jaws, mouth, lips, your cheeks, and cheekbones . . . your nostrils . . . your eyes and eyeballs, eyelids, eyebrows, the space between your eyebrows . . . temples . . . forehead . . . relax your whole head and focus your attention on your breath as if your whole body is breathing, from head to toe, and from toe to head, like one big wave, without jerks, without pauses . . .

THE "CORPSE JOURNEY" AND "BLUE STARS"

Now, bring your attention to the center of your forehead . . . prepare yourself for a grand journey in your body . . . the corpse . . . bring your attention to the center of your forehead and visualize a blue star or a bright circle (*bindu*) there . . . if you like, repeat your mantra while remaining aware of the star throughout the journey . . . let the mantra vibrate with the bright star . . . once again, in the center of your forehead, the bright star, the vibration . . . in the pit of your throat . . . the bright blue star in the right shoulder joint . . . elbow

. . . wrist . . . the tip of your right thumb . . . tip of your index finger . . . middle finger . . . ring finger . . . little finger . . . in the right wrist joint . . . elbow . . . right shoulder . . . blue star in the pit of your throat . . . the left shoulder joint . . . elbow . . . wrist . . . tip of your left thumb . . . tip of your index finger . . . middle finger . . . ring finger . . . little finger . . . in the left wrist joint . . . elbow . . . left shoulder . . . blue star in the pit of your throat . . . with each breath, feel the radiance, the vibration . . . in the heart center . . . your right breast . . . heart center . . . your left breast . . . heart center . . . your navel . . . pubis . . . perineum . . . blue star in your right hip . . . knee . . . ankle . . . in the tips of your toes from the little toe to the big toe . . . your right ankle . . . knee . . . hip . . . blue star in the perineum . . . your left hip . . . knee . . . ankle . . . in the tips of your toes from the little toe to the big toe . . . your left ankle . . . knee . . . hip . . . blue star in the perineum . . . your navel . . . heart center . . . in the pit of your throat . . . your mantra, its vibration, and light . . . blue star in the middle of your forehead with the mantra . . . the rise and fall of your breath . . . feel the breath vibrate in the whole body, in all the points, from the top of your head to the tips of your toes and from the tips of your toes to the top of your head . . . feel all the stars at the same time . . . the light and vibration, everywhere . . . like one single presence, vibrating and luminous . . . the energy points in one single field, one star . . . no pauses in your breathing . . . like a never-ending wave, allow your body to breathe through all the points . . . allow it to radiate with light and vibrations . . .

THE MOON

Bring your attention back to the contact of your nostrils with the air . . . the feeling, the movement . . . like two rays of white light . . . like the moon . . . as if your face is becoming an unblemished moon . . . a bright moon rises in the back of your throat . . . your whole face is an unblemished moon . . . your breath, two luminous rays . . . that come and go from the middle of your forehead . . . the moonlight flows through your nostrils . . . through your fingers . . . a cool and vibrating light . . . flowing through your hands like the light flowing through your fingers, as if your breath is flowing downward into your toes . . . the same light is flowing through your feet and encircling them . . . rays of light, of moonlight, flowing through your toes . . . all your agitation and physical, emotional, energetic, and mental tensions are cleansed by this cool moonlight . . . observe the moon rising in the back of your throat, your face is a disc, an unblemished moon . . . your breath, two rays . . . your hands, fingers, feet, and toes spread the moonlight . . . observe the radiance . . . taste the vibrations . . .

COMING BACK TO SITTING POSITION

Very slowly, allow the light from your hands and fingers to come back to your face . . . bring your hands to your face as if to unite the two rays . . . slowly, open your eyes filled with this light and look at your hands . . . massage your face, your temples, and the nape of your neck with your fingers full of light . . . repeat your mantra . . . sit up slowly, with awareness of the moonlight in your face, breath, hands, and fingers . . . then join the light in your hands with the light in your feet and toes . . . gently place your hands on your feet so that the rays of light unite, so that the light in the fingers and in the toes becomes one single ray of light . . . very slowly, massage your ankles, feet, and toes, and sit in any meditation pose . . .

MEDITATIVE BREATHING

Sit in any meditation pose with a straight back . . . all your limbs are completely relaxed . . . place your right hand turned upward in your left palm, at the level of the lower abdomen . . . your thumbs are touching . . . be aware of the flow of light and vibrations that unite . . . feel the luminous circle around your body . . . the moonlike disc in your face . . . the bright stars, all together, in the circle . . . the vibration of the mantra . . . feel the contact of the air in your nostrils with the mantra . . . feel the breath without pauses . . . the ray of sunlight coming out of the right nostril . . . the moonbeam entering the left nostril . . . three times . . . then the other way around . . . the moonbeam coming out of your left nostril . . . the ray of sunlight entering your right nostril . . . three times . . . then both nostrils at the same time . . . three breaths . . . that unite in the center . . . with your mantra . . . the moonbeam coming out of the left nostril as you exhale . . . the ray of sunlight entering the right nostril as you inhale . . . three times . . . then the other way around . . . three breaths . . . then feel the breath in both nostrils at the same time . . . simultaneously, uniting in the axis . . . three times . . . then exhale the sunlight through the right nostril . . . inhale the moonbeam through the left nostril . . . three times . . . then the other way around . . . three breaths . . . then observe the moon on the left, the sun on the right . . . let them unite in the middle . . . observe the breathing on both sides, without differentiation . . . between your eyebrows down to the space between the nose and the upper lip . . . with the mantra, exhale the ray of sunlight . . . inhale the moonbeam . . . feel the stars in your body . . . light, vibration . . . the circle of light all around it . . . the moon in your face . . . the flow of breath, the rays of light, the mantra . . . be silent, be still . . . a being of light . . . slowly open your eyes . . . repeat the mantra . . . total awareness of being a being of light . . . join your hands in front of your chest and bow your head . . . feel love in your heart . . . the energy in your hands . . . feel full of peace, joy, gratitude . . . chant the sound *AUM* three times . . . like a prayer . . . then go back to your activities with this feeling, allowing the light of consciousness to illuminate every moment . . .

SESSION 2
Contemplation of the Elements (*Mahabhuta Visarga Yoga Nidra*)

If one meditates on the subtlest elements in one's own body or of the world as if they are merging one after another, then in the end the Supreme (Goddess) is revealed.

VIJNANA BHAIRAVA TANTRA, VERSE 54

This fundamental practice is elementary, if I may say so, and of capital importance in learning how to navigate within the different states of matter, consciousness, and joy of being. It is a wonderful practice for recognizing the different structures of the being and going deep into the surrender and peace that result from the feeling of dissolution. It is also a practice related to falling asleep and preparing for death, with the transition from one state to another, going back to the source. With regular practice it is possible to increase the time for contemplation, meditating for up to two hours on each element. Let us note that this type of practice usually starts in the base center (the earth element generally corresponds to the base energy center); but in this session we will start in the heart center, thus going directly to a more subtle level from the very beginning, and insisting on the importance of feelings, sensations, touch, flavor, and joy. One can find traces of such practices in tantric Buddhist schools, and in the samkhya and yoga traditions, in the writings of Goraksha, such as the *Goraksha Shatakam* or, more recently, in the teachings of Sri Anirvan. This practice offers a direct path to knowing oneself, to joy without object, to the joy of being nothing and everything at the same time. As in the case of all sessions, it is recommended to begin with a meditative walk or a series of poses, gestures, and breathing exercises in direct relation with the energy centers corresponding to this particular practice.

The Practice

PREPARATION

Lie down on your back in corpse pose (*shavasana*) with your arms and legs away from the body, palms facing upward, feet turned outward, straight back . . . close your eyes . . . prepare yourself to be completely still during the whole session . . .

RELAXATION

Become aware of your general state . . . of the floor on which you are lying . . . of the distant sounds outside and of the inner sounds that are closer . . . become aware of the rise and fall of your breathing and extend your attention to the places where your body is touching the ground, from your head to your toes . . . allow the body, the shava, to rest and relax to the rhythm of your breathing, which comes and goes like waves on a tranquil ocean . . . the wave rises from your toes to the top of your head as you inhale . . . and falls from the head to your toes as you exhale, all the way down your spine . . . enjoy the feeling, the caress, the sensation that envelopes you . . . let the wave wash away your preoccupations, worries, and physical and mental tensions with each exhale . . . let yourself be enveloped by this presence . . . the waves come and go as feelings, emotions, and thoughts, but the deep ocean remains perfectly still . . . a witness of the rise and fall . . . Let yourself be filled with prana and with life every time you inhale, like gas filling your whole body . . . with a deep feeling of surrender every time you exhale . . . feel yourself enveloped in energy and vibrations . . . feel your spine vibrate when you inhale (with the mantra *SO*) and when you exhale (with the mantra *HAM*) . . . then bring your attention to the heart center and feel the energy spreading everywhere . . . feel at peace . . . enjoy the feeling that arises . . .

WISH OR RESOLVE

From the heart center and feeling the energy, with full awareness of the vibrations in the body, breathe in, hold your breath and repeat your wish three times . . . then forget it, as you exhale . . . simply observe the sensations in the body as it breathes . . . be a mere witness of the ebb and flow . . . (*SO'HAM*) . . . be completely still and tranquil . . .

ROTATION OF CONSCIOUSNESS

Bring your attention to your right thumb . . . become aware of the skin, flesh, and bones . . . feel the vibration . . . feel your index finger . . . middle finger . . . ring finger . . . little finger . . . the palm of your hand, the back of your hand . . . your whole hand . . . wrist . . . feel your whole wrist . . . and continue to your forearm . . . up to the elbow . . . your elbow . . . upper arm up to the shoulder . . . your shoulder . . . and your whole arm . . . the tissues, vibration . . . then bring your attention to your right big toe . . . second toe, third toe, fourth, and fifth . . . the sole of your foot, your whole foot . . . heel, ankle . . . enjoy the feeling . . . and allow the caress to move up to your calf . . . shin . . . knee . . . feel your knee . . . thigh, right buttock, your right hip . . . your whole right leg . . . the flesh, the vibration . . . the sensation extends to the left big toe . . . second toe, third toe, fourth, and fifth . . . the sole of your foot, your whole foot . . . heel, ankle . . . calf . . . shin . . . your knee . . . feel your knee . . . thigh, left buttock, left hip . . . your whole left leg . . . into the left thumb . . . be aware of the skin, flesh, and bone . . . feel the vibration of the image . . . your index finger . . . middle finger . . . ring finger . . . little finger . . . the palm of your hand, the back of your hand . . . your whole hand . . . wrist . . . your upper arm . . . up to the elbow . . . your elbow . . . the upper arm up to the left shoulder . . . your whole shoulder . . . and your whole left arm . . . the tissues, vibration, image . . . now feel both your arms at the same time . . . both your legs at the same time, your hips . . . allow the awareness to embrace the entire bottom half of your body . . . right and left buttocks . . . perineum, anus, coccyx . . . groin . . . the sexual and sacral region . . . tissues, vibration, image . . . and allow the awareness to go up into the stomach, plexus . . . lumbar region . . . right and left kidneys . . . to your ribs . . . then into the thoracic and dorsal regions . . . right breast, left breast . . . right side, left side . . . right and left shoulder blades . . . in between the shoulder blades . . . collarbone . . . feel both your legs, the trunk of your body, all the way to your shoulders . . . your arms . . . allow the awareness to come to your neck, throat, the nape of your neck, cervicals . . . then in your whole head: feel your nose (right and left nostrils), your tongue and mouth (upper and lower lips, your teeth), both your eyes and the space between them, the skin of your relaxed face, your ears . . . your whole head, your skull, your brain . . . the fontanel breathing . . . and feel your whole body . . . breathing in and out (*SO'HAM*), vibrating . . . observe and simply enjoy this state (listen to the mantra repeating itself naturally within you) . . . let yourself go completely with each exhale and melt into the peace in the background, a column of attention, the light of energy . . . that sees everything . . . and welcomes all phenomena that appear and disappear, without commentary, without words . . . observe the thoughts that come and go . . . without being affected by them . . . the body is sleeping but the awareness is alert . . . like a child falling asleep in its mother's arms . . . the body is sleeping but the mother is watching over it . . .

COUNTDOWN

Get ready for the countdown . . . breathe in, 108 . . . breathe out, 108 . . . breathe in, 107 . . . breathe out, 107 . . . breathe in, 106 . . . breathe out, 106

. . . continue the countdown at your own pace down to 0, to the center of yourself, to your heart . . . with each exhalation, abandon yourself to this tranquil background . . . in which the countdown appears and disappears . . . with each exhalation, go deep into this joyous silence . . . into this peaceful stillness . . . be the witness, a spectator to everything that appears and disappears in the realm of awareness . . .

CONTEMPLATING THE FIVE ELEMENTS

Earth

Now, allow your attention to completely rest in the heart center . . . with a feeling of your whole body, the earth on which it is resting . . . as a whole . . . without words and thoughts, just the feeling and the vibration . . . breathe in and become aware of the feeling of solidity, of touch . . . breathe out with a profound feeling of stillness and peace . . . (*LAM'LAM* or *SO'HAM*) . . . continue this until you have the impression of being one with the earth . . . deep contemplation, from the heart center . . .

Water

Allow your attention to come back to the throat center as you exhale . . . the transition from solid state to liquid state . . . breathe in with the awareness of the vibrant energy center . . . breathe out and let it flow in all the meridians of the body and six feet around it . . . with a deep feeling of fluidity and bliss . . . awareness of the center as you breathe in, like a bright white moon and allow the rays to flow as you exhale . . . awareness of the rise and fall of the vibrations . . . (*VAM'VAM* or *SO'HAM*) . . . continue this until you feel that you are one with the water element . . . deep contemplation, from the throat center . . .

Fire

Now allow your attention to go up to the energy center in the palate, at the back of the head, as you exhale . . . the transition from the liquid state to the fire state . . . awareness of the vibration as you breathe in, of the heat and light in the energy center . . . a deep feeling of irradiation as you exhale . . .

(*RAM'RAM* or *SO'HAM*) . . . let the fire burn the sense of form . . . the sense of "me" . . . let the fire burn desires and fears . . . do this until you feel that you are one with the fire element . . . deep contemplation, from the center of the palate . . . let the flame of attention illuminate everything that appears and disappears, breath after breath . . . all the sensations, emotions, thoughts, and images that appear and disappear . . .

Air

As you exhale, allow the attention to go up to the energy center in your forehead, between your eyebrows . . . from the fire state to the gaseous state . . . awareness of the vibration in the energy center as you inhale . . . a deep feeling of expansion as you exhale . . . of all-encompassing and formless energy, spreading throughout the universe . . . (*YAM'YAM* or *SO'HAM*) . . . as if you can touch, feel, and penetrate everything at the same time . . . without words, thoughts, images, just the feeling . . . do this until you feel that you are one with the air element . . . until you have a global and impersonal feeing of expansion, an all-embracing and impersonal energy expanding and penetrating the whole universe, free as a bird, beyond the limits of your skin and of your mind . . . allow this energy to embrace and penetrate the whole universe . . . to spread beyond all limits . . . a deep feeling of expansion . . . of dissolution . . . of being, of awareness and profound joy . . . become one with the most subtle quality of the air element . . . deep contemplation from the forehead center . . . experience the consciousness of being as you inhale, and the joy of being as you exhale . . . feel love and kindness . . .

Space

Now, as you exhale, let your attention go up to the fontanel, to the space above your head . . . (*HAM'HAM* or *SO'HAM*) . . . like the pale and clear moonlight . . . let the feeling of expansion reveal the stillness of the being in which this very feeling appears . . . the link with falling asleep, the transition . . . toward contemplation of the sky . . . of space . . . beyond forms, feeling, and thoughts . . . beyond everything . . . feel "I am," without words, thoughts . . . in absolute silence and stillness . . .

The "Two Spaces"

Be a witness, a spectator . . . when you breathe in (*SO*), be aware of the flow of vibrations coming down into the heart center . . . when you exhale (*HAM*), allow the flow of vibrations to go up from the heart center to the throat center, the palate, then to the center of the head, until its course ends in the fontanel, in the empty space . . . after each exhalation, the pause, the void, the transition . . . contemplate this movement for a few minutes, this subtle rise and fall that appears and disappears in the void . . . until you feel that the empty space in the heart and the empty space in the head are only *one* . . . above, below, and all around, there is only the total void of the infinite sky . . . the great silence in which everything appears and disappears . . . like the clouds in the sky . . . clarity, void, immense joy, without object . . . the heart, the sky of awareness . . . infinite . . . [long pause] Who is seeing? Who am I? Who does this experience and these thoughts come to? [very long pause] . . .

WISH

In this deep silence, in this vast void . . . feel the first vibration, the presence . . . and in the pause after you inhale, repeat your wish three times . . . and once again, forget about it, as you exhale . . .

FINAL PHASE

Feel the vibration, heat, and light . . . the rise and fall of the breath, coming back to revitalize the body . . . without moving . . . let the vibration of life appear once again . . . the heat, light, vibrations . . . in your head . . . in your neck . . . arms . . . trunk . . . legs . . . increase the intensity of your breath . . . enjoy the sensation of the flesh and of the vibrations, of the sound and light, of the life operating in the whole body . . . progressively, take your time and allow the body to move, starting with your fingers . . . your toes . . . arms and legs . . . Take the time to taste, to feel, with your eyes open wide. Take the time to simply stay silent, in the awareness and joy of being. Let this luminous presence illuminate your activities.

SESSION 3

From the Sound *AUM* to Non-contact
(Pranava Asparsha Yoga Nidra)

OM is the bow and the soul is the arrow, and That, even the Brahman, is spoken of as the target. That must be pierced with an unfaltering aim; one must be absorbed into That as an arrow is lost in its target.

MUNDAKA UPANISHAD,
SECOND *MUNDAKA*, CHAPTER 2:4

This session is inspired by one of the most ancient practices. It uses the sound *AUM* to stop the mind and allow the grand silence of the Self to reveal itself. Yoga nidra has roots in Kashmir Shaivism as well as in Vedic traditions. Some trace it back to the practice of asparsha yoga, the yoga of non-contact, nonrelation, and nonunion, a direct path to complete surrender, prior to all forms, systems, and states. If contact (*sparsha*) is cause for suffering, non-contact (*asparsha*) is its extinction, its liberation, where only joy remains. In his *Karika*, Gaudapada uses this term to describe Pure Awareness, the much talked about fourth state. Just as the sky is not affected by the passing clouds, the Self remains free of everything happening in it. In order to recognize this, the yogi must let go of feelings, emotions, thoughts, images, desires, and fears. In practice, it is the awareness of contact with the objects of perception that will gradually reveal the space of this non-contact. As Gaudapada says, "All fear stops when it approaches, in it there is no more fear, but only divine peace, eternal illumination, an invariable and unchanging absorption. There is nothing more to give or take, not even the slightest fear remains. At that time, the eternal knowledge will set in itself, in Atman, remaining the same and going to sameness." In other words, it is the perception of phenomena that reveals the awareness that one can have of the ineffable. The practice uses sound to reveal the silence and uses a support to recognize that which is without support, or *contactless,* the awareness and joy without object. The term *asparsha yoga* is an oxymoron that stops the dualistic fluctuations of the mind, in order to reveal its nonduality. It is the yoga of self-inquiry that looks directly at what hides behind every desire and effort, including the desire to be free. The essence of this yoga is not an action, for there is nothing to do. There is simply being. This means practicing each session with joy and ease, without prehension. Here are the guidelines of this type of session.

The Practice

PREPARATION/RELAXATION

Sit down in a meditation pose and relax your body from head to toes, part by part (see session 1, page 103); be aware of the physical body. Then, being totally aware of every breath, go up from the toes to the head, taking your time to feel the vibration, especially at the level of the energy centers along the spine; be aware of the energetic structure. Feel the vibrations in the whole body and bring your attention to the heart center as a witness of all phenomena that appear and disappear . . .

AUM CHANTING

Be attentive and chant the *AUM* sound eighteen times, feel the vibration climbing up from the heart center, to the throat center, to the forehead center, and finally disappearing in the void above the head . . . be aware of the empty pause after each exhale, after each chant . . .

MOVE INTO LYING-DOWN POSITION

Staying totally aware of each breath and of the vibrations in the body, lie down in corpse position, observe the transition from one pose to the other . . . make your body completely still . . . bring your attention to the heart center . . .

observe . . . (you can also breathe in, hold your breath, repeat your wish three times, and forget it, as you exhale) . . .

ROTATION OF CONSCIOUSNESS WITH THE SOUND *AUM*

With each breath, repeat the sound *AUM* mentally, remaining aware of the vibration in each finger of your right hand, starting with the thumb . . . in your wrist . . . elbow . . . shoulder . . . your whole arm . . . the sound *AUM* vibrates in each one of these points . . . in each toe of the right foot . . . in your right ankle . . . knee . . . hip . . . your whole right leg . . . repeat the same in your left leg . . . in your left arm . . . then feel the sound and vibration in your perineum, in the base center . . . in the sacral region and the center of your pubis . . . solar plexus, lumbar spine, navel center . . . in the heart center, radiating in the chest and dorsal spine . . . in the throat center, in the cervicals . . . in the center of your head . . . in your whole body, in the axis . . . just the sound, the feeling, vibrations everywhere . . . allow this subtle feeling to embrace and spread out to the whole universe . . .

AUM AND EFFACEMENT

Bring your attention back to the heart center . . . continue to mentally chant the sound *AUM* . . . be aware of the silent space in which the sound appears and disappears . . . witness the mind as it repeats the mantra . . . until the sound and the mind completely fade away in this silent void . . . in this silence that you are . . . either you stop the chant and merge with the silence . . . or you allow the sound to stop where it rises and falls . . . [long pause] . . . if thoughts arise, be aware of the distraction without appraising it, and once again start repeating the sound *AUM* until it subsides into silence . . . keep doing this as long as it is necessary . . . Who is chanting *AUM*? . . . Observe this . . . with practice, these moments of silence and pure meditation will become longer . . .

FINAL PHASE

(You can breathe in, hold your breath, repeat your wish three times, and forget it, as you exhale) . . . once again, be open to the silent space and chant *AUM* mentally . . . with the rise and fall of your breath . . . and be aware of the sound and the vibration in your whole head . . . in your neck . . . shoulders and arms . . .

chest and back . . . in your stomach . . . hips . . . the base of your trunk . . . your legs . . . feel your whole body, alive and vibrant . . . and come back to any sitting meditation position, observe the transition from one pose to the other . . . stay still and chant the sound *AUM* out loud one last time . . . then open your eyes . . . and remain attentive to the silence that is always present, beneath the sound . . .

> *O Goddess, meditate on the AUM sound, rising from the heart center (A), to the throat center (U) and then to the center of the head (M), until it merges with the silent Void above.*
>
> INSPIRED BY THE *VIJNANA BHAIRAVA TANTRA*, VERSE 39

SESSION 4

The Art of Dying (*Marana Yoga Nidra*)

> *One should meditate on one's own fortress (the body) as if it were consumed by the Fire of Time, rising from the foot. At the end (of this meditation) the peaceful state will appear.*
>
> *Meditating in this way by imagining that the entire world has been burnt, a person whose mind is undisturbed will attain the highest human condition.*
>
> *VIJNANA BHAIRAVA TANTRA*, VERSE 52–53

> *Whosoever, at the end, leaves the body, thinking of any being, to that being only he goes, because of his constant thought of that being.*
>
> *Therefore, at all times, remember Me, and fight, with mind and intellect fixed (or absorbed) in Me; you shall doubtless come to Me alone."*
>
> *BHAGAVAD GITA*, 8:6–7

This session addresses the theme of death, to force us to face our human condition. The perception of our finiteness can strengthen the awareness of life expressing itself in the present moment. When thoughts are stopped, I can only admit that I know nothing; therefore, death is just another belief among others, like a concept. In the absence of projection and fear, and in this stillness of the body and the mind, the joy of being is revealed in all its splendor. During one's personal practice, this session can last for the time it takes for a corpse to burn, which is approximately three hours. One's attention should always come back to sensations so that the visions do not become thought associations, but only serve the experience, which will also burn in the space of nonrelation, non-contact, and free of object (asparsha). It is advised to practice the session related to the elements (session 2, page 108), before this one, with a tension-free body, and a happy and peaceful mind. With practice, these two sessions will merge in the experience of a unique path toward silence. Moreover, as the *Vijnana Bhairava Tantra* indicates, the dissolution of the body can further spread to the dissolution of the whole universe, until the joy of being nothing reveals itself to be the joy of being everything.

The Practice

PREPARATION

Perform a series of postures, breaths, gestures, and concentrations to ignite the fire of sensations, as if for the very last time . . .

"DRAMATIZATION* AND RELAXATION"

Lie down on your back . . . inhale, tighten your arms and legs, as if the whole body is stiffening, hold your breath while tightening the whole body and being aware of the shava, then exhale forcefully and let everything go . . . [repeat

---

*Read the section "Sleep and Death" beginning on page 43 about death and the experience of Ramana Maharshi.

three times] . . . observe the whole body relaxing . . . your eyes are closed, arms and legs away from the body becoming more and more still with each breath . . . as if it was dead . . . ask yourself, without looking for an intellectual answer, "Who is dying?" . . . witness the shava . . . motionless, peaceful . . . inhale, life . . . exhale, death . . . be aware of the last breath, of the empty pause after exhale . . . every time you breathe out, let go of the tensions in the body and in the mind . . . every time, go deeper, withdraw into the heart center . . . after every exhalation, the pause, the transition . . .

WISH

In this profound tranquility . . . breathe in, hold your breath, repeat your wish three times, and forget it as you exhale . . .

ROTATION OF CONSCIOUSNESS

(read session 2, page 108) . . . Bring your attention to all the points of fire—thumbs, toes, eyes . . .—to the energy centers in the joints and along the axis, and be aware of the heat, light, vibrations, radiation, and fire in the body . . .

COUNTDOWN

(read session 2, page 108) . . . To go deeper into the unknown, into the nonknowing, feel the empty pause, the transition between wakefulness and sleep, between life and death . . . let every sensation, emotion, thought, and image dissolve in the tranquil background . . . effortlessly . . .

CREMATION

(If you have been to Varanasi, and/or if you are inspired by this place, you can now visualize or imagine yourself at Manikarnika Ghat, the renowned cremation ground, on an unlit pyre . . . and welcome the feeling that this image brings up . . .) Be aware of the still body and mind . . . as if they were dead . . . your family members and your friends are paying their respects . . . when you were born, the people around you were laughing, perhaps now, they are crying . . . observe this scene and the feeling it brings up in you . . .

be a witness, an equanimous spectator . . . as if you are watching a movie . . . then imagine fire near your feet . . . listen to the crackling . . . feel the warmth under your soles . . . the sacred fire is the light of consciousness, beyond the world of projections . . . the flame of vision, of attention . . . let the fire kindle your right toe . . . feel the glowing ember, hot and vibrant in your right big toe . . . then let the fire of time and the feeling spread to both your feet . . . feel the flame of sensations irradiate and spread with the rise and fall of your breathing . . . in your heels . . . ankles . . . calves . . . like two incense sticks, slowly burning . . . feel the purification of the sacred fire, the burning love that cleanses and dissolves . . . as the flames rise, feel the burnt parts falling to ashes . . . disappearing . . . let the fire burn your knees, it is getting more and more fierce . . . in your thighs up to your hips . . . sensations, vibrations . . . the fire is burning more intensely . . . allow the body, the image of the body and all its resistances fade away . . . disappear . . . your arms, starting with your thumbs . . . the base of your trunk continues to burn slowly . . . the fire climbs up the spine . . . with the rise and fall of your breathing, of sensations . . . the anus, pubis, navel, heart, neck, head . . . your whole body is on fire, burning . . . falling to ashes . . . fire and breath that erase everything . . . feel the warmth that has spread all around, beyond the fire itself . . . feel the light of the fire in the space all around . . . in all directions at the same time . . . until all sensations fade away . . . the whole body is burnt, fallen to ashes dispersed by the wind . . . ashes to ashes, dust to dust . . . only *that which is* remains . . . neither the body nor the mind, only Presence remains . . . joy, silence, peace, and transparence of empty space . . . (let the purifying fire spread to the whole world and the entire universe . . . to other bodies, to cities, forests, mountains, and planets . . . until they are all completely burned to ashes, until nothing of the phenomenal world remains . . .) . . . feel "I am" even when there is nothing . . . neither form, nor feeling, nor thought, nor word, nor image . . . feel that even before thinking "I am dead or alive," "I am" . . . silence and peace . . . eternity . . . being . . . consciousness . . . bliss . . . empty and full at the same time . . . [long pause]

WISH

In this profound tranquility . . . inhale, hold your breath, repeat your wish three times, and forget it as you exhale . . .

FINAL PHASE

Slowly, bring your attention back to the phenomena that appear in your conscience . . . remain the witness of the "I" thought and of the sense of "me" . . . of the whole universe . . . the galaxies, the sun, the planets, the Earth, different bodies . . . of your own body . . . the image, the breath, the vibrations and sensations from head to toe . . . life coming back once again, into all your cells . . . feel alive and vibrant . . . allow the silence to enter every cell of your body . . . feel the joy of being . . . the awareness of being . . . and with this taste, breathe deeply, start to slowly move your body . . . stretch your limbs, yawn and come out of yoga nidra, with the impression that you are under a broader gaze . . . feel purified, empty, vacant, transparent, free, and glowing with kindness and love for all beings . . .

115 Practices to Inspire and Create Your Sessions

Although obvious and simple, recognizing the Self is not an easy matter. It depends on the sensitivity of each individual. This is why so many paths, schools, and "techniques" exist, each one representing an endeavor to identify the most important thing. Thus, we can also compose a session with different bases for concentration or angles of observation. The *Vijnana Bhairava Tantra* mentions 112 "micro-practices" that one can address separately, in a direct way, during the day or at night.* These

---

*I have referred to 115 verses as 115 micro-practices, even though three of them (verses 69, 70, and 106 in the *Vijnana Bhairava Tantra*, corresponding to numbers 46, 47 and 83 in this book) do not directly mention a concentration. Therefore, logically, we come to 112, which corresponds to the number mentioned in the tantra (verse 39). But we can also consider that the concentrations 21–22, 88–89, and 110–111 are each one micro-practice, among other possible combinations.

practices can also inspire yoga nidra and its sessions, in a gradual manner, addressed separately or developed and combined together (read sessions 2 and 4, pages 108 and 118). They highlight intuition, the stopping of the mind, fullness, bliss, spatiality, effacement, presence, beingness, *shivaitness,* energy, void, and nonduality. If knowing God is the only goal, then attention is the means par excellence to recognize God, especially when the attention awakens to itself, beyond dualistic thoughts, after having "stumbled" during one of these attempts, in between two states.

With the help of the micro-practices mentioned below, and using the previously mentioned sessions as inspiration, you can compose an infinity of long or short yoga nidra sessions. For example, you can start with the relaxation phase, possibly the resolve or wish, the rotation of consciousness, and the countdown, before focusing your attention on one or several of the following concentrations:

1. Be aware of the inhaling breath that descends and the exhaling breath that ascends, and of the two voids, inside and outside, where the breaths appear and disappear.*
2. Meditate on the voids between inhalation and exhalation, then between exhalation and inhalation.
3. Stop the breath and thoughts in order to reveal the Space where the two voids meet.
4. Meditate on the energy of the retained breath either inside (with full lungs) or outside (with empty lungs).
5. Meditate on the luminous and radiant energy rising from the base center until it dissolves in the empty space above the head.
6. Meditate on the rising energy in the form of lightning as it

---

*Vijnana Bhairava Tantra. The first practice mentioned here is inspired by the twenty-fourth verse. Therefore, the second practice corresponds to the twenty-fifth verse, and so on.

moves upward from one center to another until it reaches the empty space above the head.

7. Allow the letters of the (Sanskrit) alphabet to vibrate in each center, from the base center, to the pubis, to the navel, the heart, the throat, in the forehead in between the eyebrows, in the fontanel, to the energy of consciousness above the head in the Void.

8. Fill the body up to the fontanel with the vital energy of breath and having crossed the fontanel like a bridge, contract the eyebrows to make the mind free from dualistic thoughts.

9. Enter the Heart of the absolute void by meditating on the voids where the five senses emerge and dissolve.

10. Bring awareness to an external object, without superimposing the mind, and allow the energy of concentration to merge in itself.

11. Fix the attention on the inner space of the skull and, sitting motionless with closed eyes, stabilize the mind.

12. Meditate on the space within the central channel that allows the energy to flow freely.

13. Block the openings of the sense organs with your hands to cut off all impressions, and perceive the light point merging in the infinite space.

14. Allow a small flame to appear in the mind's space, between the eyes, then concentrate on it in the space above the head and in the heart center until it disappears in the void.

15. Meditate on the uninterrupted sound that vibrates in the heart center and that is perceived by the ear, and let the supreme beatitude carry you away.

16. Meditate on the *AUM* sound, rising from the heart center (*A*), to the throat center (*U*), and then to the center of the head (*M*), until it merges with the silent Void above the head.

17. Meditate on the silent space at the beginning and at the end of the uttering of any letter.

18. Listen attentively to the sound of a musical instrument until it melts into silence, and merge with it.

19. Visualize any letter and hear its sound, then allow the image and the sound to merge with the vibration of the void.

20. Meditate on the void in the body and all around, from all sides, simultaneously.

21. Meditate simultaneously on the void above and on the void at the base.

22. Meditate simultaneously on the void above, on the void in the heart, and on the void at the base in order to stop all thoughts.

23. Once the mind is still, feel the void in any place in the body.

24. Meditate on all the elements constituting the body as pervaded by void.

25. Meditate on the body as only enclosed by the skin with nothing inside, until the One that cannot be meditated upon reveals itself.

26. Merge the senses in the space of the heart, until joy bursts forth.

27. Meditate on an empty space or on the void in the whole body.

28. Concentrate on the empty space of the heart or the fontanel, always and everywhere.

29. Meditate on the body as if it were consumed by fire from head to toe, until only the ashes, dispersed by the wind, remain.

30. Meditate with an undisturbed mind, imagining that the entire world has been consumed by flames.

31. Meditate on the subtlest elements in the body or of the world as if they are merging one after another, until the Original Consciousness is revealed.

32. Feel the energy of the breath, dense, subtle, and loud, in the space of the fontanel, then enter the heart at the time of sleeping, to be aware of dreams and sleep.

33. Meditate on the entire universe dissolving progressively in the void of the subtlest forms.

34. Perceive the reality of Shiva, up to the ultimate limit, in all forms of the universe.

35. Imagine the whole universe as being a void and let the mind completely dissolve in it.

36. Be aware of the empty space in any vessel while paying attention to its enclosing walls.

37. Contemplate any vast space devoid of all objects for a long time, and let your thoughts dissolve there.

38. Meditate on the space between two objects, states, thoughts, breaths, and so on, and rest in that space.

39. Be aware of the still attention that has abandoned one object, and that immediately moves on to another object.

40. Feel that the body and the whole universe consist of nothing but Consciousness.

41. Be aware of the meeting of the two breaths in the void, and of the complete harmony.

42. Feel, contemplate, and taste the whole body and the whole universe as being filled with bliss.

43. Welcome the beatitude and reality that are revealed by the trick of tickling oneself.

44. Close all the openings of the sense organs, feel the prickly sensation produced by the upward rising of the energy of breath, and let supreme joy burst forth.

45. Be aware of the expansion of sexual energy and joy during sexual intercourse.

46. Attentively observe the orgasm with full awareness of the energy in the body.

47. Even alone, recall with awareness the moment before the orgasm and the flood of pleasure.

48. At the time of experiencing great happiness, or the joy of seeing a friend or a relative after a long time, meditate on the rising of this happiness.

49. Be aware of the pleasure that emerges while eating or

drinking (meditate on the pleasure and not on the object of pleasure).

50. Meditate on the joy obtained from music and art in general.

51. Be aware of the feeling of satisfaction and its relation with supreme bliss.

52. Concentrate on the moment of falling sleep and on the moment between waking and sleeping states.

53. Direct the gaze to a space filled with the light of the sun, the moon, or a lamp.

54. Be totally aware of the moments where the "me" dissolves: the body is lying flat on the ground, as if dead, in the corpse pose; the energy of the body in a moment of anger, the unwavering gaze and attention; the uninterrupted moving of the lips and concentration on the taste; the tongue turned upward and contemplation of the void.

55. Meditate while sitting on a seat, maintaining hands and feet without any support.

56. Sitting comfortably or lying down, place the arms in a curved position and fix the mind on the void under the armpits.

57. Fix the gaze without blinking on an external form and make the mind supportless.

58. Keeping the tongue in the center of the mouth wide open and concentrating on the soft *h* sound as I inhale and exhale, allow the mind to be dissolved in peace.

59. Sit on a seat or lie on a bed and meditate on the body as being supportless.

60. Be aware of the slowness of a moving vehicle or of the moving body and flow in the tranquility of the flood of consciousness.

61. Contemplate the cloudless and clear sky for a long time, without blinking or moving the body.

62. Contemplate the whole sky as if it is Shiva, and let it pervade the head until it is perceived in all things.

63. Be aware of the nature of Shiva in the waking, dream, and deep sleep states, as the common substratum of these three states.

64. Meditate on the darkness outside, on a dark night.

65. Meditate with closed eyes on the inner darkness, allowing the mind to dissolve there, and then meditate with open eyes on the darkness outside and recognize the common space in which all this appears.

66. When an accident or deliberate obstacle obstructs the function of a sense organ, be aware of the nondual state of void.

67. Chant or recite the *A* sound, without ending in a nasal or aspirated sound.

68. Fix your awareness with a mind free of any support at the end of the aspirated *H* (*visarga*) of a letter.

69. Meditate without any support by feeling the body in the form of the vast sky, unlimited in all directions.

70. Concentrate on the pain that appears when a part of the body is pierced with a sharp object or needle.

71. Perceive the void of the mind, of the intellect, and of the ego.

72. Observe all phenomena and realize that it is always dualistic thought that separates them, thus creating the illusion of duality.

73. Observe a desire as it arises spontaneously and put it to rest immediately, so that it merges in the very space from where it has sprung.

74. Feel that "I am" even before the arising of will and knowledge, and simply remain as "Being."

75. Once knowledge and will have arisen, fix the mind on the point where they emerge, free of all object.

76. As soon as the desire arises to know an object or to know about something, fix the mind on the space of knowledge itself.

77. Recognize that the same Consciousness is residing in billions of bodies, transcending time.

78. Be peaceful in the various states of desire, anger, greed,

intoxication, or jealousy, and meditate on the silent background in which these states appear.

79. Contemplate the whole universe like a mere spectator or as if it were a movie show, without identifying with it.

80. Observe the game of pleasure and pain with attention and equanimity, without getting caught up in it.

81. Unidentified with the body, realize that "I am everywhere" and blissful.

82. See that knowledge, desire, and activity appear in oneself and in all objects simultaneously and melt into their common and omnipresent substance.

83. Be aware of the unity beyond all dual relations between subject and object.

84. Experience the consciousness in the body of others as well as in one's own body, feeling the consciousness of every being as one's own consciousness.

85. Free the mind of all support, of all thoughts, and spontaneously recognize the nonduality of the Self.

86. Because I am omniscient, omnipotent, and all-pervading, recognize that I am not different from Shiva and that I am Shiva.

87. Realize that all phenomena spring from oneself, just as waves arise from water, flames from fire, and rays from the sun.

88. When one falls to the ground with exhaustion and the energy of agitation comes to an end, taste that state of availability.

89. Be attentive to all moments of the loss of consciousness, when the mind disappears.

90. With open eyes and without blinking, remain attentive to the inner and outer spaces at the same time.

91. Closing one's ears and similarly closing or contracting the anus, listen to the inner sound.

92. Stand above a deep well or an abyss and let all thoughts dissolve in the depth.

93. If the presence Shiva is all-pervading, where else can I go?

94. Use each impression of the sense organs to recognize the peaceful consciousness in which everything appears.

95. Use the moment of sneezing, or when fear or sorrow appear in a moment of catastrophe or surprise, hunger, or thirst, to recognize the essential reality.

96. When the thought of a remembered object appears in a familiar place, welcome it and let it dissolve here and now, in the pure awareness of the body.

97. Fix the gaze on a particular object, then slowly withdraw the gaze, as well as any thought of the object, until one becomes an abode of the void.

98. Meditate on the energy of consciousness that emerges from intense devotion.

99. Look at an object and all other objects surrounding it as if they are in the same fields of perception, and meditate in the peace of this empty and impersonal space.

100. Be free of thoughts of purity and impurity by becoming aware of the joyous gaze, free of the thoughts that it illuminates.

101. Know that nothing exists apart from Consciousness.

102. Be happy in peace without form and equanimous in all situations.

103. Be free of desire and aversion, and in the space in between them, be Pure Awareness.

104. Recognize the unknowable, the ungraspable, and the all-pervading void as Shiva himself.

105. Contemplate the space, supportless and free from limitation, and recognize and merge with the nonspace, beyond beingness and nonbeingness.

106. Fix the attention on an object, only to withdraw it immediately, thus leaving the thoughts without any support in the empty space that contains them.

107. Chant the name of Bhairava until one is identified with Shiva.

108. While making assertions like "I am this or that" or "this is

mine," remember that before being this or that, "I am," and find the supportless peace.

109. Meditate on words such as *eternal, omnipresent, without any support, all-pervading, and Lord of All That Is* until one attains fulfillment in accordance with their meaning.

110. In order to obtain peace, consider the whole universe as an illusion.

111. Perceive clearly that external objects depend on the knowledge of one's senses and one's mind, and that beyond this limited perception, in the Vision of the Self, the whole universe is void.

112. See that there is neither bondage nor liberation beyond the fear, and that the universe is reflected in the mind just as the sun is reflected in water.

113. Recognize that all pleasure and pain occurs through the senses, in order to be detached from the senses and abide within the Self.

114. When attention awakens to itself, contemplate knowledge and the known as being only One.

115. When the vital energy, the mind, the individual consciousness, and the limited self have disappeared, recognize the true nature of Shiva.

After a long silent pause, you can repeat your wish (if you made one at the beginning of the session) and then finish the session as is indicated in the examples given before. You can also practice these techniques spontaneously, at any time of the day or night, without any specific preparation.

Let us understand well that it is not about progress, nor stages, nor accumulation, nor doing anything, when it comes to realizing Consciousness. Deep knowledge of even one of these concentrations is enough to taste the nondual silence of the Self and wisdom, after the fluctuations of the mind have been stopped. This is why the practice essentially consists in continuous contemplation, remembering the Self, during the day or at night. It is to this remembering that these practices lead us, as do rituals, prayers, or the natural mantra of the breath (*HAM'SA, SO'HAM,* "I am"). True meditation is only about remaining in this still and permanent presence, without effort and without agitation. It is also the heart of yoga nidra.

APPENDIX

"The Taste of Yogic Sleep"

An Interview with Pierre Bonnasse

From *Le Journal du Yoga* 160

Q: Where does yoga nidra come from?

PB: From Lord Narayana himself! Yoga nidra is mainly transmitted orally, and it would be impossible to know its precise and exact origins in time. Ancient texts mention it by referring to Vishnu in eternal repose. Popular illustrations show Shiva in the corpse pose. The *Mandukya Upanishad* lays the foundations for yoga nidra. In his commentaries, Gaudapada, Shankaracharya's master's master, mentions a form of non-contact yoga (*asparsha yoga*) that is linked with yoga nidra. Gaudapada's master is supposed to have been Narayana himself. In the end, everything comes from the self and returns to the self, and there is only silence.

Q: Can you describe the technique of yoga nidra for our readers?

PB: As a means, yoga nidra deploys a variety of practices for waking up, during the day, when we fall asleep at night, and during the night. There are preparatory techniques that include different postures, breathing exercises, and concentrations for observing these processes and awakening to a finer quality of attention. And there are also the regular long sessions that are practiced, motionless, in the corpse pose. They begin with a relaxing one's body, followed by observing one's breath, bringing a subtle awareness of the physical, energetic, and mental structures. It all depends on the intention. The session can further explore the different structures of the being, the different states of consciousness, the transitions and the interval, the senses, desires, fears, the mind's process . . .

Q: How important is the energetic structure in this practice?

PB: Particularly important, because it allows one to understand the connections that the energy structure has with the body and the mind. There are many sessions that explore the functioning of the chakras (energy centers), *nadis* (meridians), and *pranavayu* (vital breaths of respiration, digestion, excretion, and so on) in relation with therapy or for knowing oneself. Tasting the energy and feeling the life that goes through us and lives in us is the door to Being and the joyous Presence to oneself.

Q: What are the important moments in yoga nidra?

PB: When yoga nidra ceases to be a technique, an action, and reveals itself to be a quality of being. When attention awakens to its own substance. When the practitioner disappears, when fear disappears and what remains is the impersonal presence of consciousness and pure joy. Then, it is no longer an "important moment," but the eternity in which all moments occur. It is grace in all its splendor.

Q: What is the connection between yoga nidra and relaxation?

PB: Relaxation is the foundation. One must be relaxed in order to go deep into yoga nidra. The more relaxed and peaceful I am, the more permeable I am, available and open to another influence. First, I must track down the tensions. If I am aware of what I am holding on to, forewarned of the mind's pattern, it is possible to let go and new degrees of relaxation will be revealed. The most subtle contractions will dissolve in the light of attention. And the one who is holding on disappears in the end. Or not! [laughs] By combining very deep relaxation with very alert watchfulness, I can recognize the ever peaceful space, which, by nature, is free from tension. And thus it is neither tensed nor relaxed. From this space, a gentle feeling of peace and liberation emanates.

Q: Could we say that yoga nidra is meditation in sleep?

PB: If you like, but it addresses the state of wakefulness as much as the dream and deep sleep states. These three states are interconnected and one cannot understand one state without understanding the others, nor can one understand these three states without recognizing the reality that unites them all. It is the taste of being without ego, a taste without object. Meditation is happening, but there is nobody to do it.

Q: What are the traditions or lineages that have influenced you?

PB: Yoga, Vedanta, and tantra. The teachings of Ramana Maharshi and Nisargadatta Maharaj have touched me deeply. On the subject of yoga, I have been greatly inspired by the teachings of Sri Aurobindo, of the natha yogis of Varanasi, Sri Anirvan, and the Himalayan Masters. But life is the greatest teacher, close to me, always available, behind every breath and in between the breaths.

Q: Is it important to follow a particular tradition or lineage?

PB: What is important is to experience tradition, allow it to flow through us. Receiving and giving teachings that have proved their worth for centuries and sharing this practice with other beings— that is essential and sacred. It is the very essence of the transmission. This tradition is eternal, without birth. Then how can it disappear? We are One with it, it is not a separate thing.

Q: What is the approach that you have presented in this book?

PB: The conciliatory one, an approach combining the important points of view (darshana) in Indian philosophy with the teachings I have received. But I try to have the most phenomenological approach possible. This calls for forgetting what one knows about things, to come back to the things themselves, to their appearing and their origin. Being a witness to the birth and the resorption of the world, at every moment. It is an approach of nonprehension. This is true for the author, but also for the reader who must take over the inner process and taste the experience, the exploration, and the void. That is where the reader will find his or her true guide, and also, the answer to your first question. [laughs]

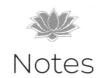

Notes

Most citations from sacred works were translated into French from the original Sanskrit by the author (and from French into English by the translator).

INTRODUCTION.
INDIAN PHILOSOPHY AND
THE LIMBS AND PATHS OF YOGA

1. Patanjali, *Yoga Sutras*, 1:2.

PART I.
THE PHILOSOPHY OF YOGA NIDRA

1. *Vishnu Sahasrnamam Stotra*, chapter 149 of the *Mahabharata*.
2. Porte, *Shiva le Seigneur du sommeil* (French).
3. Sarah Combe, *Un et multiple, Dieux et déesses, mythes, croyances et rites de l'hindouisme* (French) (Dervy, 2010).
4. Adi Shankaracharya, *Yoga Taravali* (Chennai, India: Krishnamacharya Yoga Mandiram, 2003) 25–26.
5. Swami Gambhirananda, *Mandukya Upanisad, With the Commentary of Sankaracarya* (Calcutta: Advaita Ashrama, 1979).
6. *Mandukya Upanishad*. Also see *Brihad Aranyaka Upanishad*, 4:3.9, 3.15. *Chandogya Upanishad*, 11:1.
7. Maharshi, *Talks*.

8. *Shiva Sutra*, part 1, verses 7 to 11. Also see Dyczkowski, *The Aphorisms of Siva*.

9. Pierre Bonnasse, *Sur les rives de Mère Ganga* (French) (Santé-Yoga Editions, 2012).

10. *Bhagavad Gita*, 13:1–2.

11. Nisargadatta, *I Am That*.

12. Anirvan, *Inner Yoga*.

13. Ibid.

14. Nisargadatta, *I Am That*.

15. Shankaracharya, *Tattva Bodha*.

16. Anirvan and Reymond, *To Live Within*.

17. *Bhagavad Gita* 2:23–24.

18. Klein, *Who Am I*.

19. *Bhagavad Gita*, 2:62–63.

20. Maharshi, *Talks*.

21. Montaigne, *Essays*.

22. Maharshi, *Talks*.

23. See www.sriramanamaharshi.org.

24. Montaigne, *Essays*.

25. *Bhagavad Gita*, 8:6–7.

PART II.
THE PRACTICE OF YOGA NIDRA

1. Nisargadatta, *I Am That*.

2. Anirvan, *Inner Yoga*.

3. Ibid.

4. Tikhomiroff, *Le Banquet de Shiva*.

5. Anirvan, *Inner Yoga*.

6. Ibid.

7. Ibid.

8. *Rig Veda*.

9. *Vijnana Bhairava Tantra*, 75.

10. Anirvan and Reymond, *To Live Within*.

11. Anirvan, *Inner Yoga*.

12. Tracol, *Pourquoi dors-tu Seigneur?* (French).

13. Anirvan, *Inner Yoga.*

14. Anirvan and Reymond, *To Live Within.*

15. Anirvan, *Inner Yoga.*

16. *Vijnana Bhairava Tantra*, 55.

17. *Brihad Aranyaka Upanishad*, 4:3.7; *Chandogya Upanishad*, 8:1.1; *Taittriya Upanishad*, 2:1.

18. Satyananda, *Yoga Nidra.*

19. *Bhavana Upanishad*, 8.

20. *Bhagavad Gita*, 6:24–25.

21. André Riehl, *Le Sommeil et le Regard de Shiva* (lecture given in French on August 15, 2006).

22. Ibid.

23. Shankaracharya, *Upadesha Sahasri*, 11.6.

24. Papin, *Siva Samhita*, 2:1–3.

25. Maharshi, *Talks.*

26. *Tantraloka*, 6:10.

27. Anirvan, *Inner Yoga.*

28. *Ashtavakra Gita*, 1:4.

29. Swami Shantananda Puri, *Jivanmukti: Liberation Here and Now* (Bangalore, India: Parvathamma C. P. Subbaraju Setty Charitable Trust, 2002).

30. Shankaracharya, *Upadesha Sahasri*, 16.8.

31. David Godman, ed. *Be as You Are: The Teachings of Sri Ramana Maharshi.*

32. Adi Shankaracharya's, *Dashashloki*, 8 and *Atma Shatakam*, 5.

PART III.
PUTTING YOGA NIDRA INTO PRACTICE

1. Swami Veda Bharati, excerpt from a conference given in Budapest, Hungary, 2010.

Suggested Readings

Publications that deal exclusively with the subject of yoga nidra are rare, even though the number of books published about yoga in general is impressive. I have listed below some references that have notably influenced me or, in one way or another, have a direct link with the teachings that are mentioned in this book.

Anirvan, Sri. *To Live Within*. 2nd ed. Sandpoint, Idaho: Morning Light Press, 2007.

———. *Inner Yoga*. Sandpoint, Idaho: Morning Light Press, 2008.

Anirvan, Sri, and Lizelle Reymond. *Le pèlerinage vers la vie et vers la mort*. Gollion, Switzerland: Infolio, 2009.

Aurobindo, Sri. *La Force du Yoga*. Selected and introduced by Pierre Bonnasse. Paris, France: Seuil, 2011.

Balsekar, Ramesh. *Pointers from Ramana Maharshi: Read and Reflect*. Mumbai, India: Zen Publications, 2008.

Bouchard d'Orval, Jean. *Reflets de la Splendeur: Le Shivaïsme tantrique du Cachemire*. Paris, France: Almora, 2009.

Buttex, Martine, trans. and ed. *108 Upanishads*. Paris, France: Dervy, 2012.

Chinmayananda, Swami. *The Holy Geeta*. Mumbai, India: Central Chinmaya Mission Trust, 1996.

———. *A Manual of Self-Enfoldment*. Mumbai, India: Central Chinmaya Mission Trust, 2010.

Dyczkowski, Mark, trans. and commentary. *The Aphorisms of Siva: The*

Siva Sutra with Bhaskara's Commentary, the Varttika. Albany: State University of New York Press, 1992.

Feuga, Pierre, trans. and commentary. *Cent douze méditations tantriques: Le Vijnana Bhairava Tantra.* Paris, France: Accarias, 2007.

Hart, William. *The Art of Living: Vipassana Meditation as Taught by S. N. Goenka.* Mumbai, India: Embassy Books, 2000.

Klein, Jean. *Who Am I? The Sacred Quest.* Oakland, Calif.: Non-Duality Press, 2006.

Lakshman Joo, Swami. *Kashmir Shaivism: The Secret Supreme.* Author House, 2003.

———. *Vijnana Bhairava: The Practice of Centring Awareness.* Varanasi, India: Indica Books, 2007.

Maharshi, Ramana. *Talks with Sri Ramana Maharshi.* Thiruvannamalai, India: Sri Ramanasramam, 2006.

———. *Be as You Are: The Teachings of Sri Ramana Maharshi.* Edited by David Godman. New York: Penguin Books, 1989.

Michael, Tara, trans. and commentary. *Hatha Yoga Pradîpikâ: un traité de Hatha Yoga.* Paris, France: Fayard, 1974.

———. *Yoga.* Monaco: Le Rocher, 1980.

Miller, Richard. *Yoga Nidra: Awaken to Unqualifed Presence Through Traditional Mind-Body Practices.* Amazon Digital Services, 2010.

———. *Yoga Nidra: The Meditative Heart of Yoga.* Louisville, Colo.: Sounds True Inc., 2005.

Montaigne, Michel Eyquem de, *The Complete Essays of Montaigne.* Translated by Donald M. Frame. Redwood City, Calif.: Stanford University Press, 1957.

Nisargadatta, Maharaj. *Consciousness and the Absolute.* Edited by Jean Dunn. Durham, N.C.: The Acorn Press, 1994.

———. *I Am That.* Compiled and translated by Maurice Frydman. Durham, N.C.: The Acorn Press, 1984.

———. *Prior to Consciousness.* Edited by Jean Dunn. Durham, N.C.: The Acorn Press, 1990.

Norbu, Namkhai. *Cycle of Day and Night.* Barrytown, N.Y.: Barrytown/ Station Hill Press, Inc., 2000.

———. *Dream Yoga and the Practice of Natural Light.* Ithaca, N.Y.: Snow Lion Publications, Inc., 2003.

Panda, N. C. *Yoga Nidra, Yogic Trance: Theory, Practice and Applications.* New Delhi, India: Printworld, 2003.

Papin, Jean, trans. and commentary. *Gheranda Samhita: Traités Classiques de Hatha-Yoga.* Paris, France: Almora, 2013.

———. *Siva Samhita: Traité Classiques de Hatha-Yoga.* Paris, France: Almora, 2013.

Patanjali. *The Yoga-Sūtra of Pantañjali: A New Translation and Commentary.* Translation and commentary by Georg Feuerstein. Rochester, Vt.: Inner Traditions, 1989.
Note: There are many good variations of Pantanjali's Yoga Sutras that could be referenced.

Porte, Alain, trans. and commentary. *Ashtavakra-Gita: Les Paroles du Huit fois difforme.* Paris, France: Editions de L'Eclat, 1996.

———. *Shiva le Seigneur du Sommeil.* Paris, France: Seuil, 1993.

Rama, Swami. *Exercise Without Movement.* Honesdale, Penn.: Himalayan Institute Press, 1984.

———. *Living with the Himalayan Masters.* Honesdale, Penn.: Himalayan Institute Press, 2007.

———. *OM the Eternal Witness.* Dehradun, India: Himalayan Institute Hospital Trust, 2007.

———. *Path of Fire and Light.* Vol. 2. Honesdale, Penn.: Himalayan Institute Press, 2007.

Rhiel, André. *Le Regard de Shiva.* Interview. France: Les Entretiens de La Falaise Verte, 2006.

Riviere, Jean M. *L'asparsha Yoga: Un yoga pour l'Occident.* Paris, France: Arché Milano, 1989.

———. *Lettres de Bénarès.* Paris, France: Albin Michel, 1982.

Satyananda, Swami. *Yoga Nidra.* Bihar, India: Bihar School of Yoga, 1980.

Silburn, Lilian, trans. and commentary. *Le Vijnana Bhairava.* Paris, France: College de France, Institut Civilisation Indienne, 1999.

———. *Kundalini: The Energy of the Depths.* Albany: State University of New York Press, 1988.

Tikhomiroff, Christian. *Le Banquet de Shiva: Pratiques et philosophie du Natha-Yoga.* Paris, France: Dervy, 2013.

Tracol, Henri. *Pourquoi dors-tu Seigneur?* Paris, France: Pragma, 1983.

Wangyal, Tenzin. *The Tibetan Yogas of Dream and Sleep*. Ithaca, N.Y.: Snow Lion Publications, 1998.

Veda Bharati, Swami. *Night Birds: A Collection of Short Writings*. Rishikesh, India: AHYMSIN Publishers, 2000.

Waite, Dennis. *Back to the Truth: 5,000 Years of Advaita*. First published by O Books, U.K.: Mantra Books, 2007.

● ● ●

For more information (additional resources, yoga teacher trainings, etc.) visit www.rishiyogashala.com and www.nidra-yoga.com (the latter is mostly in French but contains some English components).

Index

BOOKS OF RELATED INTEREST

The Heart of Yoga
Developing a Personal Practice
by T. K. V. Desikachar

The Path of Modern Yoga
The History of an Embodied Spiritual Practice
by Elliott Goldberg

The Yoga-Sūtra of Patañjali
A New Translation and Commentary
by Georg Feuerstein, Ph.D.

The Yin Yoga Kit
The Practice of Quiet Power
by Biff Mithoefer

Chakras
Energy Centers of Transformation
by Harish Johari

Awakening the Chakras
The Seven Energy Centers in Your Daily Life
by Victor Daniels, Kooch N. Daniels, and Pieter Weltevrede
Illustrated by Pieter Weltevrede

Tantric Kali
Secret Practices and Rituals
by Daniel Odier

Fasting the Mind
Spiritual Exercises for Psychic Detox
by Jason Gregory

INNER TRADITIONS • BEAR & COMPANY
P.O. Box 388 • Rochester, VT 05767
1-800-246-8648
www.InnerTraditions.com

Or contact your local bookseller